Praise for Conquering Your Child's Chronic Pain

by LONNIE K. ZELTZER, M.D., and CHRISTINA BLACKETT SCHLANK

"This is an important, compassionate book that offers a mind-body-spirit approach to helping children and their families emerge from suffering and find joy in life."

>   —*Deepak Chopra, author of* Fire in the Heart

"Parents! If you have a child in pain, read this book. There is hope. Pain in children is surprisingly common and a source of much misunderstanding and anguish. Many treatment options exist for your child, and this book thoughtfully presents the many options available."

>   —*James Campbell, M.D., professor of neurological surgery and director, Blaustein Pain Treatment Program, Johns Hopkins University School of Medicine; founder and president, American Pain Foundation; past president, American Pain Society*

"Dr. Zeltzer and Ms. Schlank have written an outstanding book for parents of children and adolescents with chronic pain. For any parent who has left a doctor's office saying to himself or herself, 'What exactly did the doctor say about why my child still has pain?,' this book will help. For clinicians and trainees, this book is an ideal refresher course on the experience of chronic and recurrent pain for children and parents and on cognitive-behavioral, psycho-educational, and rehabilitative approaches to treatment. I recommend it highly."

>   —*Charles Berde, M.D., Ph.D., chief, Division of Pain Medicine, Department of Anesthesiology, Perioperative, and Pain Medicine, Children's Hospital, Boston; professor of anesthesia and pediatrics, Harvard Medical School*

"This thoughtful book by one of the pioneers and leading thinkers in the area of chronic pain in children provides, in a clear and concise way, the background information that parents need to understand what is going on with their sons and daughters and offers practical strategies to ameliorate their discomfort. It offers parents techniques that they can use and markers by which they can evaluate progress. This is a valuable and important book that will be appreciated by every family struggling with a child in pain."

—*Neil L. Schechter, M.D., professor of pediatrics, University of Connecticut School of Medicine; director, Pain Relief Program, Connecticut Children's Medical Center*

"Dr. Zeltzer draws upon years of experience as one of the world's leading authorities on pediatric pain treatment in writing a book that parents will find reassuring and informative. Parents will gain hope when they discover the many available treatment options. The book is easy to read and provides sympathetic and realistic advice, especially to those who have pursued the often long and frustrating search for help. Pediatricians also will find the book a helpful resource when caring for children who suffer from chronic pain."

—*Kenneth R. Goldschneider, M.D., F.A.A.P., director, Division of Pain Management; associate professor of anesthesia and pediatrics, Cincinnati Children's Hospital Medical Center and Susmita Kashikar-Zuck, Ph.D., associate professor of pediatrics, Psychology Division, Cincinnati Children's Hospital Medical Center*

"*Conquering Your Child's Chronic Pain* is not only an interesting work but an exciting presentation. I am particularly touched by her experiments and research on yoga as practiced by me, which she says has wonderful effects on these children. Asanas and breathing techniques work on the organic and nervous systems and regulate the hormonal secretions by the glands. This yoga works on their psychology by building courage and confidence and inspiring children to develop healthy minds. I hope Dr. Zeltzer continues to do such subjective research on yoga so that the young generation regains freedom from pain and can lead positive and dynamic lives."

—*B.K.S. Iyengar*

"A wonderful book! Dr. Zeltzer's approach is loving, respectful, upbeat, and—best of all—successful. *Conquering Your Child's Chronic Pain* will be required reading for the staff of many pediatric pain clinics, including ours at Duke, in addition to being highly recommended for the parents of the children we serve."

—*Laura Schanberg, M.D., associate professor, pediatric rheumatology, Duke University Medical Center*

"Although it is written for parents, I would highly recommend this book to all medical practitioners who treat children and adolescents with pain problems. If pediatricians and family practitioners read Dr. Zeltzer and Ms. Schlank's book, they would fill their palette of treatment options for many patients in their practices. Most importantly, this book offers parents hope and much practical advice on treating many different pain problems. It is a must-read for any patient with chronic pain."

—*Steven J. Weisman, M.D., Jane B. Pettit Chair in Pain Management, Children's Hospital of Wisconsin; professor of anesthesiology and pediatrics, Medical College of Wisconsin*

"Dr. Lonnie Zeltzer is a pediatrician who uses leading-edge science, drugs, and complementary medicine to help her patients at her UCLA clinic to conquer pain. Now her wisdom is available to all."

—*Patrick J. McGrath, O.C., Ph.D., F.R.S.C., Canadian Institutes of Health Research Distinguished Scientist; Canada Research Chair; Killam Professor of Psychology and professor of pediatrics and psychiatry, Dalhousie University*

"This book is grounded in top-level scientific and clinical expertise on the biomedical and psychological aspects of children's chronic pain. Yet it is easy and accessible. The style is clear and captivating, with vivid examples drawn from varied real-life situations. This is an amazingly caring, competent, and useful book. It opens your mind but also your heart, and it gives you effective means to be of real help to the suffering child."

—*Vanna Axia, Ph.D., professor of developmental psychology, Child Neuropsychiatry Specialization School, School of Medicine; director, Graduate Program in Developmental Psychology, University of Padova, Italy*

Conquering Your Child's Chronic Pain

Conquering Your Child's Chronic Pain

A Pediatrician's Guide
for Reclaiming a Normal Childhood

LONNIE K. ZELTZER, M.D.
and
CHRISTINA BLACKETT SCHLANK

A HARPERRESOURCE BOOK
An *Imprint* of HarperCollins*Publishers*

HarperCollins books may be purchased for educational, business, or sales promotional use. For information please write: Special Markets Department, HarperCollins Publishers, Inc., 10 East 53rd Street, New York, NY 10022.

FIRST EDITION

Designed by Mary Austin Speaker

Library of Congress Cataloging-in-Publication Data

Zeltzer, Lonnie K.
    Conquering your child's chronic pain : a pediatrician's guide for reclaiming a normal childhood / Lonnie K. Zeltzer, and Christina Blackett Schlank.
        p. cm.
    Includes bibliographical references and index.
    ISBN 0-06-057017-2
        1. Pain in children.   2. Pain in adolescence.   3. Pain—Psychological aspects.   4. Chronic pain.   I. Schlank, Christina Blackett.   II. Title.

RJ365.Z45   2005
    618.92'0472—dc22

                                                            2004054353

---

05   06   07   08   09   WBC/RRD   10   9   8   7   6   5   4   3   2   1

{ TABLE OF CONTENTS }

{ ACKNOWLEDGMENTS }

This book was born out of my wish to share all that I have learned and observed over more than 30 years as a pediatrician, a clinical specialist caring for children with chronic pain, and as a researcher. I have learned much from my valued colleagues in this emerging field of pediatric pain, including those with expertise in pediatric functional bowel disorders. I appreciate their willingness to share their wisdom and experience in this book.

I thank my fellow faculty members in the Pediatric Hypnotherapy Workshop for the Society for Developmental and Behavioral Pediatrics. You have taught me how to be playful and have fun while teaching.

Thanks also to my staff, faculty members, and fellows in the UCLA Pediatric Pain Program for their willingness to take on the load of clinical, educational, and research work while I was at home writing and writing. I especially thank my patients and their parents for sharing their knowledge and experience in order to help others.

I thank Diane Bass, L.C.S.W., and writer-director Jane Segal for their many interviews of families. I also appreciate the help I received from Beth Sternlieb (Iyengar yoga teacher), Manouso Manos (Iyengar master), Allison Woolery (UCLA psychology graduate student), Sean Hampton, M.P.T. (physical therapist), Esther Dreifuss-Kattan, Ph.D. (art therapist and psychoanalyst), J. Kathryn de Planque, Ph.D. (hypnotherapist), Michael Waterhouse, M.S., L.Ac. (acupuncturist and Chinese herbalist), Colleen Werner, R.N. (biofeedback specialist), Diane Poladian, P.T. (biofeedback and physical therapist), Chris Slate (craniosacral therapist), Cynthia Myers, Ph.D. (psychologist and massage therapist), Erin Wilson (massage therapist), Audrey Easton, Ed.D., and Carolyn Coleridge, M.S.W. (energy therapist). I thank Sherry Dunay Hilber for her help on humor and pain. I also thank my meditation teacher, Trudy Goodman, for help in writing about mindfulness, as well as Dr. Steve Weisman, for his mindfulness meditation instructions for parents. Thanks also to Stanford student Jennifer Hsiao and my daughter Carin Zeltzer, who researched Web sites for the book (and Carin for helping me with many computer jams!).

I appreciate the help of Kathy Allameh on the book and for the kindness and professionalism she showed every day coordinating with our patients and our team. Dr. Leah Ellenberg's help with the neuropsychological information is also appreciated. Caryn Freeman helped with all of the information about school. (Also, thanks to Laura Hale, Assistant Principal, Sherman Oaks Center for Enriched Studies.)

I also especially appreciate the patience and expertise of my cowriter, Christina Schlank, who spent time in our pain clinic and read voluminously. She did this all in the latter months of her pregnancy. If that isn't a tribute to mothers, I don't know what is! Thank you, Myles, for your patience with us! This book would not be what it is without Christina's creative abilities and excellence in writing. This truly was a collaborative effort in all senses of the word.

Thank you also to my editor, Toni Sciarra, whose clarity of mind and gentle hand helped preserve the spirit of this book. And many thanks to my most supportive agent, Madeleine Morel.

I am indebted to my parents, Laura and Garry Kaye, for encouraging my curiosity as I grew up. Especially, thanks to my mother for her many phone calls asking me repeatedly, "So what are you writing about again?" I appreciate my sisters, Deana Luchs and Andrea Goldberg, and my brother Glenn Kaye, who helped explain and reexplain to our mother what I was writing about.

I believe that children teach their parents, and this certainly has been the case for me. I have learned much from our very bright, loving, and creative daughters, Shira, Alysa, and Carin. They contributed to this book before I even began to write it. Their guidance, patience, wisdom, and great sense of humor helped nurture me in the writing process and added sparkle to my thoughts. I am truly indebted to them and love them very much. I also want to thank my son-in-law, Neil Goldman, for his wonderful sense of humor, warmth, and creativity, all of which found their way into this book.

Finally, no words can adequately express my appreciation for the love, support, and wisdom that I have received from my husband, Paul. Throughout our 35 years together, he has been the source of my strength, and it is to him that I dedicate this book with my deepest love and affection.

{ PROLOGUE }

A Mother's Story About Living with Her Son's Chronic Pain

Our teenage son, Ted, had suffered from muscular pain since the age of two, but as he entered adolescence, the pain had become so debilitating that he had to withdraw from school when he was 13. In a special program, he was schooled at home for 10 months with a tutor, until he became unable to do any work at all because he was either in too much pain or too dulled from the medications. We had seen every specialist, every expert, read all that we could get our hands on, and still our son had to endure terrible pain, was unable to sleep until he was finally just too exhausted to stay awake, and often made statements about just wanting to die instead of having to live this way. Our frustration had mounted to astronomical proportions because every doctor contradicted every other doctor. We left every consultation with the parting advice that Ted would just have to "live with it" because there was no cure. We were all overcome with feeling helpless and hopeless.

* * *

I first heard about Ted when I was called by the patient coordinator at the University of California, Los Angeles (UCLA), who asked me if I treated children who have pain that no one else has been able to "fix." Whenever someone asks me that, I always wonder whether the patient's attitude has gotten to the "No one else has cured me, so why should I trust that you can?" stage.

Not that I fear this kind of response; to the contrary, I look at it as a challenge. I feel that surge of energy that comes from knowing you will be able to help someone where others have failed. What made me anxious is that I was told that the mother of this boy had fibromyalgia and that she and her son were giving each other Demerol injections at home. The woman from the insurance company who had contacted the UCLA patient coordinator indicated that she believed that both were drug addicted. I was actually worried about seeing this family and wondered if my team and I would be able to help this boy.

* * *

By the time Ted was admitted to the Pediatric Pain Management Program at UCLA, he was requiring three to four Demerol injections per day, muscle relaxers, and hydrocodone (Vicodin). Even with all that, he was still in miserable pain, depressed, and completely removed from his once-busy teenage life. At our first consultation and examination at UCLA by Dr. Zeltzer and psychologist Dr. B, we were informed that not only did Ted have fibromyalgia but he also had a pain anxiety disorder and his brain was constantly giving him messages that he was in pain, which increased his anxiety, which fueled his pain. That was the bad news.

* * *

I was surprised when I finally met with Ted that the problem was not as complex as I was led to believe. On the basis of the story that I heard from the insurance company case manager, I was expecting the family to be resistant to any type of treatment that took effort. It was clear that the insurance person with whom I spoke not only did not like this family but was angry with them for "creating problems." That is, she thought that they (mom and son) were both making up their pain in order to get drugs, and the insurance company "didn't want any part of that." This "faking pain for drugs" is not an uncommon complaint that I hear when patients are referred to me. To my delight, Ted's family was motivated to work to improve the situation for their son, and they all had a great sense of humor.

• • •

The good news was that the doctors were very confident that they could help Ted. It was the first flicker of hope that we'd been given in our search. So we began the journey. . . .

• • •

It was clear that Ted had fibromyalgia, low self-esteem, and feelings of helplessness, and that he had anxiety that was also driving his pain. He was sensitive and often felt the conflict between his parents and was especially attuned to their different styles of parenting and how they responded to him. Because his mom also had fibromyalgia, she identified with his suffering. That made it more difficult for her to see him suffer, causing her to behave in ways that Ted's dad viewed as much too solicitous.

Ted was relying on the Demerol because he saw medication as the only thing that gave him some relief, although he admitted that it reduced his anxiety and helped him sleep rather than actually reducing the pain. What became clear to us in our evaluation was that Ted would need to enter our eight-week intensive inpatient pain rehabilitation program. During Ted's stay, we expected that he would learn coping skills and enhance his self-esteem by learning to function in spite of his pain, which would then lessen the pain. He would also be observed so that he could receive appropriate medication to help him wean off the opioids and address his anxiety in less drug-related ways. And he would learn biofeedback; undergo occupational, recreational, and physical therapy; and receive acupuncture treatments. He was in for a lot of hard work!

However, because pain is a family affair, we would not admit him into our program unless both parents agreed to participate. This meant intensive couple/parental and family therapy, often several days per week, for the entire hospital period. Despite the fact that his parents lived almost three hours from the hospital, they were determined to work to improve things for the entire family. And did they ever work!

•   •   •

It has now been one year since Ted's completion of the UCLA pediatric pain program. I am amazed at how accustomed to normal life we've become. Ted is a confident, happy, healthy 15-year-old, with no resemblance to the young boy whose every waking moment was filled with pain and hopelessness. Today he is strong-willed, noisy, and overflowing with testosterone-laced energy. Just the way we like it.

There Is Light at the End of the Tunnel

Pain is no evil unless it conquers us.
—GEORGE ELIOT

I can hardly believe that until the late 1980s it was commonly accepted in the medical world that children do not feel pain in the same way that adults do. In fact, during my training, it was common practice to rationalize that infants do not feel pain, but that even if they do, they don't remember it. So it was that infants underwent major surgery without anesthesia and no postoperative pain medication. Often they would be given a medication that would paralyze them but leave them fully aware of the pain.

I remember learning to perform circumcisions on newborns during my pediatric training while they were strapped to what was called a papoose board. I watched, horrified, as their little faces turned beet red and they screamed their heads off. I remember asking my supervisors whether the babies needed something for their pain; they reassured me that the babies were just crying from the stress of being restrained and that they really didn't feel the pain. This medical "truth" was always offered to me with more than a little condescension. In those days, there were few women in medical school, and the not-too-subtle message was that if I was too squeamish, then maybe I shouldn't be in this field.

During my pediatric residency in the early 1970s, there was a 10-year-old boy on my service who had a tumor that had spread throughout his body. He did not make eye contact and just whimpered. The team would make rounds with the attending oncologist, who would show the residents how to identify skin nodules and an enlarged liver and spleen, using this boy as a human guinea pig. My fellow residents poked and prodded him as he continued to whimper. His mother stood helplessly by and tried to comfort him. No pain medication was offered. I couldn't concentrate on what I was being taught and kept wondering what he was feeling and how he withstood such abuse. The attending physician was a very caring doctor; but the current party line was that it was "bad" to give strong painkillers such as narcotics to children. He was just practicing state-of-the-art medicine back then.

Medical thinking did not begin to change until the late 1980s after several studies were published in scientific journals showing that even the youngest children—premature babies—experience pain. In fact, babies may be more sensitive to pain because the parts of their nervous system that control pain are not fully developed. We also know that significant early pain experiences can actually have a big effect on the developing nervous system, cause children to become more sensitive to pain, and may contribute to the development of chronic pain later in life.

Whether pain is labeled "acute" or "chronic" can be rather arbitrary. Typically, pain that continues for three months or more is considered "chronic pain," and any pain lasting less than that is called "acute pain." Still, there are certain types of pain that are classically considered "acute." Examples include pain after surgery, trauma-related pain (e.g., breaking an arm), or pain related to a procedure like a blood draw or immunization. In this sense, *acute* means that most children get over this type of pain in a relatively short amount of time. However, there are some children for whom pain will continue beyond the time frame expected for most children. For these children, the pain becomes persistent, or ongoing.

For example: A child falls and suffers a minor ankle sprain. Two weeks later the child has severe pain in the sprained area, the area is supersensitive to touch, and the child can no longer walk on that leg. Even though it has been only two weeks and not three months since the initial accident, the child's severe symptoms would suggest that the pain has become chronic and will need immediate intervention so that it doesn't get worse or spread to other areas of the body. Even though the acute injury has likely healed, the child's pain-signaling apparatus has been "turned on" and something is stopping the signals from being "turned off," stopping the body from returning to normal.

In this case, as in most cases of chronic pain, treatment would be aimed at helping the body's natural pain control system to start working effectively again. (It's important to remember that the injury has healed, but the body's pain system has malfunctioned.) In upcoming chapters, I explain how, specifically, this happens.

Children's nervous systems are still growing and changing until early adulthood, and it is never too late to treat pain in children no matter how long it has lasted. This is good news for parents of children with chronic pain, who often may feel hopeless and helpless. Try to remember this when some unevolved doctor tells you that "there is nothing further that can be done" and that your child will just have to "learn to live with the pain." This is total nonsense! I don't doubt that some doctors believe these statements, but they are simply false.

So why a book specifically on pediatric chronic pain? There is certainly much written on adult chronic pain, but why children? Pain is a serious problem in one of every five children and adolescents in the United States, according to the American Pain Society. And chronic pain stems from a wide range of conditions.

Consider these statistics.

- Of U.S. children aged 5 to 17 years, 20% suffer chronic headaches.
- Twenty percent of children complain of stomach pain at least three times a week for a period of at least three months at a time.
- Juvenile arthritis (JA), one of the most common chronic diseases of childhood, affects as many as 200,000 to 300,000 U.S. children.
- The prevalence of fibromyalgia in children has been estimated to be as high as 6% in school-age children. (The actual prevalence may be higher because in many children with fibromyalgia, the condition is not accurately diagnosed.)
- Recent evidence suggests that a high percentage of children and adolescents with Asperger's syndrome and autism spectrum disorders also have chronic pain.
- In 2010, 1 of every 1,000 U.S. children will be a survivor of childhood cancer.
- Each year, 1.5 million U.S. children have surgery, and many of them have inadequate pain relief. For about 20%, the pain becomes chronic.

Chronic pain can impact all aspects of a child's life, including school attendance and grades, participation in sports and other activities, and interaction with family, friends, and others. The way a child experiences and reacts to chronic pain is influenced by many interrelated factors such as age, personality, ability to cope, activity level, anxiety, and previous experiences with pain.

In addition, children's responses to questions about how much pain they feel can be influenced by fear of, or trust in, the individual asking the question, by whether they think their answer will lead to an injection or an excuse from school, and by fatigue or emotions. How children cope and function in the face of pain is also influenced by many different factors, such as self-doubt or self-confidence, feelings of control, and even how their parents respond to them.

Children and their families experience significant emotional and social consequences as a result of pain and disability that can last for years. We know that there are genetic, psychological, and environmental contributors to the development of chronic pain syndromes, such as fibromyalgia, muscle pain, headaches, and abdominal pain (and for children with irritable bowel syndrome, associated symptoms such as diarrhea, constipation, nausea, bloating). We also know that the physical and psychological changes that go along with growth and development in childhood make the understanding and treatment of pain in children different than in adults. This is why pain programs created for adults often are not successful in treating children with chronic pain.

What I find most fascinating is that despite a relatively high prevalence of chronic pain in children and its substantial physical, psychological, social, and economic impact on children and their families, it is often underrecognized and undertreated by clinicians. In fact, until recently, chronic pain was viewed as a symptom of something else, not as a separate condition. This is why during my medical training, I was taught to approach pain by looking for the diseases and other conditions that could be causing the pain. If none were apparent, then you were forced to conclude that the child was just faking it to get attention or that there was an underlying psychological cause, and you referred the child to a mental health professional. This approach has never felt right to me.

Even today, many physicians still use this outdated model to diagnose pain. Fortunately, however, the field of pain medicine has made tremendous strides in recent years, and there are national (e.g., American Pain Society, American Pain Foundation) and international (e.g., International Association for the Study of Pain) societies that have been success-ful in educating clinicians and researchers. Hospitals now must provide a system of documentation of pain assessment for all patients before accred-itation is given or continued. In some states, such as California, the med-ical licensing board is now requiring 12 hours of CME (continuing medical education) credits for education in pain and palliative care, al-though it doesn't require education in pediatric pain per se.

Before we begin this pain journey together, it might be helpful for you to know something about my interest not only in chronic pain but also in the connection between mind and body in the healing process. This in-terest began in my undergraduate years in college and followed a cir-cuitous path to my ultimate choice of a career dedicated to treating children with pain, teaching others to understand pain in children, and ex-tensive research in pediatric pain.

In college, while I was a premedicine major, I took a number of psychology, anthropology, and sociology courses. The more I learned, the more I became fascinated by the role of the mind, including thoughts and emotions, in physical well-being. I read about other cultures in which shamans and other spiritual healers had powers to impact well-being and even illness by what they said, as well as through herbs and various rituals. My growing interest in the connection between the mind and body and its role in physical and emotional health further invigorated my desire to be-come a physician.

I applied to medical school at a time when few women were ac-cepted. In fact, in my medical school class of 100 students, I was one of four women. (There were two women in the class before me, and none be-fore that.) During the summer between my first and second year of medical school, another student and I were accepted into a psychiatry department summer fellowship. What influenced me the most that summer was my contact with the anthropologist Dr. Margaret Mead, who was a visiting fellow that summer. Her stories about her observations and experiences with traditional peoples convinced me that the path medicine had taken in our industrial world was missing something—the understanding and willingness to harness the power of the mind and beliefs to heal.

I began to search for a medical specialty in which I could explore this new (to me at least) paradigm or way of thinking about healing more fully. While I had originally intended to become a psychiatrist, that summer's experience with Dr. Mead convinced me that pediatrics would offer me the greatest opportunity for affecting the health and well-being of people through their earliest experiences, when their nervous system, mind, beliefs, emotions, and body were still developing.

I was particularly drawn to adolescents at that time, because many changes take place during those years on both emotional and physical levels as the child transitions from childhood to adulthood. (Adolescence used to be defined as ages 13 to 18, but now it is more like ages 11 to 25.) I began to volunteer in the adolescent medicine clinic at my medical school. The more time I spent with adolescents, the more intrigued I became by symptoms of suffering, such as pain, nausea, vomiting, and itching. I also became fascinated by how the developmental process of adolescence influenced the outcome in disease. Unlike during infancy, another period of rapid growth and development, adolescents can talk about their thoughts and emotions, and I found this extremely exciting.

I decided to become a pediatrician with a subspecialty in adolescent medicine. After my pediatric residency and a year as a "pediatric consultant locum" in London, I completed an adolescent medicine fellowship. During that training experience, I spent time caring for many adolescents and I became focused on those with chronic disease, especially those whose adolescence got in the way of their disease. (What I mean by "got in the way of their disease" is that because adolescence is a period when teenagers are being bombarded by inner changes and outside stresses, they are particularly sensitive emotionally and physically, and they tend to experience everything, including pain, more intensely.) This is when I first developed a real passion for discovering and understanding the symptoms of suffering. Thus I began my clinical and research interest in chronic pain, which continues today.

My research likewise continued to expand. In the 1980s, I studied the medical uses of hypnosis for treatment of pain and cancer treatment–related nausea and vomiting. I later began to study the pain-control effects of other nontraditional therapies in children, such as Iyengar yoga, acupuncture, and meditation. With Edith Chen, who was a UCLA psychology graduate student at the time, I studied the impact of children's memory on their experience of pain. These earlier studies led to a program of research that has focused on understanding why some children develop chronic pain and how to alter that trajectory. The goal is to develop ways to prevent children from ever developing chronic pain. My program's research also has been examining the role of puberty, hormones, and cognitive and emotional factors in the development of chronic pain, as well as why females develop more chronic pain syndromes, such as fibromyalgia, migraines, and irritable bowel syndrome, than do males, especially beginning during adolescence.

Eventually my clinical and research interests merged at UCLA when I arrived in 1988 to develop a pediatric pain program. For the last 16 years, I have focused almost entirely on chronic pain in children of all ages, including those youth transitioning into young adulthood. Additionally, my interest and experience with mind–body medicine has also grown during this time. Today, the UCLA pediatric pain clinic has developed into a truly integrative program that combines conventional medical practices, physical therapy, and psychotherapy with complementary therapies such as acupuncture, hypnotherapy, Iyengar yoga, biofeedback, massage, art therapy, and energy healing.

During my many years of treating children with chronic pain, I have learned much to share with you. As a parent of three daughters, I wish that I had known when they were younger what I now know about pain. One of the things that I have learned is that there are some common ways of reducing suffering in children with very different chronic pain conditions, including irritable bowel syndrome (IBS), migraines, tension headaches, fibromyalgia, complex regional pain syndrome (or CRPS, previously called reflex sympathetic dystrophy, or RSD), musculoskeletal (myofascial) pain, cancer-related pain, arthritic pain, and other pain disorders.

It is always amazing to me that children who have chronic pain, often for such long periods of time, and who have gone through so many evaluations by different subspecialists and diagnostic tests and treatments, have conditions that seem to me fairly easy to understand and treat, if the right framework is used and the right questions are asked. With the help of the information in this book, you can become an advocate for your child and obtain the most effective treatment for your child.

One of the most distressing aspects of my role as a physician during my career has been witnessing the frustration and helplessness of parents who are thwarted in their attempts to find treatment for their child's pain. Sadly, every year thousands of parents are told by their child's physician either that there is nothing physically wrong with their child or that there is nothing that can be done medically to relieve the pain—and in almost all cases, neither of these statements is true. Meanwhile, parents must watch as their children endure debilitating chronic pain day after day.

I see these children and their parents in our clinic every day. The children come from a range of cultures and socioeconomic groups. Some are highly educated; others are not. They come from single-parent households and two-parent homes. Some children have severe psychological problems; others appear to have none. They are of all ages, shapes, and sizes. Their symptoms and the degree of pain they experience differ wildly. But what connects all these children is that the pain, regardless of what it stems from, is keeping them from living normal lives.

Children who suffer from chronic pain don't have the luxury to be children—they spend a lot of time worrying, being afraid, and sitting in doctors' offices. None of us would want this for our child. I wouldn't want this for my children. But most parents of suffering children simply don't know what else to do.

Throughout the many years that I have been treating children with chronic pain and their parents, I am always struck by the degree to which parental guilt is tied up in the pain. Parents often feel guilty for their behavior. "I work too much," "My husband and I fight too much," "We shouldn't have moved out of our old neighborhood—she was so happy there." These are all sentiments I have heard again and again from parents. Or parents blame themselves for the extent of their child's pain or how long it has affected their child. "I didn't recognize the pain early enough." "I didn't believe her when she said she was in pain." These are all typical feelings.

Early on in my practice, I suspected that the guilt stemmed from what, for parents, is the ultimate sense of helplessness—watching a child suffer. As parents, we naturally blame ourselves when our child is in pain and we can't make it go away. However, though it is true that what we say and what we do—or don't do—can affect a child's perception of pain and ability to heal, these are most often not the source of the pain. As a parent myself, I am keenly aware of the guilt and other emotions associated with simply being a parent—even of a healthy child. But as a doctor treating children with chronic pain, I see how that guilt can spread and infect many aspects of family life, especially in families in which a child has been suffering with pain for a prolonged period.

For example, parents who feel guilty because their child is suffering may become overprotective, inadvertently hindering their child's ability to overcome the pain. I say this not to give parents something else to feel guilty about but rather to point out how pervasive and destructive guilt can become. I hope to give you the tools to recognize and get rid of this unnecessary feeling.

Pain does not affect just the child. Chronic pain moves into the home and invades the whole family—it exacerbates marital stresses and sibling rivalries. The child with chronic or recurrent pain begins to feel out of control, and parents feel helpless. Although most parents learn how to parent by using their own life experience and common sense, pain often seems to defy both these tools.

Parents often fear that they "missed something serious" and that the pain is a signal that there is something terribly wrong with their child that can cause irreparable harm or even death if not properly diagnosed and treated. Thus, when doctors conduct tests and say that they can't find anything wrong, parents may not know what to do next. Should they take their child to more doctors for more tests? Should they change doctors? Should they seek alternative therapies? If so, which ones? These are all important questions addressed throughout this book.

Most parents I see desperately want to know what is wrong with their child. In short, they want a diagnosis. Often a diagnosis is possible, such as CRPS, IBS, or some other disorder. However, a diagnosis is only a part of the equation, and some parents of children with chronic pain are frustrated by a lack of a concrete label for their child's pain. I completely understand: If there is a diagnosis, then there might be a cure, a magic pill that will make it all go away.

However, for most chronic pain conditions, there is no magic pill. By the time the pain has become "chronic," it has multiple factors that keep it going, add to its strength, and contribute to functional disability associated with the pain. Pain takes on baggage as it gains strength—to stop it, all the baggage must be identified, disentangled, and dismantled. This job is a joint effort on the part of the clinicians, the child, and the parent, not something to be done by the doctor alone. However, it is natural that most parents want to be able to visit the doctor and have the doctor present them with a diagnosis and then simply give their child a medicine that will work immediately and completely; have no side effects, and require no effort on the part of the child or family. Why not? That's what we all would like!

Living with a child in pain is difficult—but it need not be unbearable. I have seen amazing family triumphs in the face of severe chronic pain. Almost without exception, the families who flourish are those who find a way to take control of the pain instead of letting it control them. I have learned a great deal from the families who have shared their lives with me as we have worked together to help their child heal. I now have the pleasure and honor to share this knowledge and experience with other parents and children.

Conquering Your Child's Chronic Pain offers you and other parents (and your child if he is old enough) a way to take control of the pain—regardless of the cause—and, ultimately, help your child to become pain free. In this book, I explain the biology and psychology of pain and detail the approaches to diagnosis and treatment that we use in our program. Children and their parents who have been or are still coping with chronic pain share stories about how they have suffered, survived, and flourished in the face of chronic pain, including what techniques they use for alleviating pain, which medications and therapies worked and which didn't, and a wide range of useful coping skills. The book also answers questions that parents and children have told me they would have liked answered when they were battling chronic pain.

Conquering Your Child's Chronic Pain will teach parents and children ways to manage and alleviate pain through breathing, muscle relaxation, and visualization exercises. Once these tools are learned, they can be practiced at home to control pain and help your child cope with pain at school or elsewhere. This book explores how children express pain and how to interpret what they say. It also gives parents resources for finding the right doctor, tips for asking the right questions, and techniques for getting an insurance company to pay for alternative treatments.

My ultimate goal in this book is to provide you with the tools to become good advocates for your child within the health care system as well as to educate you about what you can do at home to help your child (and, as a result, make your family life better).

My hope is that this book will become the ultimate handbook for parents of children who suffer from a wide range of chronic pain problems, from stomachaches and muscle pain to cancer-related pain and pain associated with developmental disorders such as autism and Asperger's syndrome. Though in this book I describe characteristics that are unique to different pain conditions, there are some underlying commonalities that pertain to all children with chronic pain. Thus, in this book you will learn how to:

- Reduce your child's central nervous system arousal
- Help your child learn to cope and function normally
- Cope as a family so that you can help your child function as well as possible
- Help your child's body heal
- Help your child develop a sense of optimism and even a sense of humor in the face of pain

I believe that with information and guidance, you, as a parent, can take on these tasks successfully and also educate your child's doctors to help you achieve your goals for your child. I can't stress enough how important it is to understand that (1) in most cases, chronic pain must be treated with some combination of drugs, complementary therapies, and education, or psychotherapy and (2) patience and a positive outlook are your greatest allies.

I share with you my own experiences as a parent and as a physician. Many of my patients and their families and my clinical colleagues also generously share with you their stories and advice from personal experience. My goal is to educate you so that you can get the most effective and efficient chronic pain treatment for your child. After you have finished reading this book, you may be surprised to learn that you know more about the topic than your child's doctor! If this turns out to be the case, please be patient with him or her. We take this journey together for the sake of our children.

PART I

Pain and Your Child

CHAPTER ONE

What Is Pain?

That which hurts, also instructs.

—BENJAMIN FRANKLIN

Mark is a 14-year-old whose gastroenterologist could not find a cause for the chronic esophageal pain he had had for four months, during which he was unable to eat, sleep, attend school, or engage in other normal activities. Mark initially had developed significant pain when swallowing, which continued until a yeast infection was diagnosed and treated. By that time, however, he had had the pain for six weeks and had missed the first month of school. After the infection was gone, his pain remained, despite a normal-appearing esophagus. Mark began spending hours during the day crying, moaning, and scratching at his chest. Instead of getting better, his pain was getting worse.

• • •

It can start quite suddenly.

Your daughter complains about a stomachache, which you attribute

to the fast food she gobbled down at dinner the night before. Soon you notice she is complaining of similar aches in her stomach every few days. A
couple of days later, you notice her limping and rubbing her leg. When
you ask her about it, she says her leg feels hot and prickly. The complaints
seem unconnected, but you take her to the pediatrician for the stomach
problems. The doctor attributes the stomachaches to nerves. "After all,"
he says, "the new school year is approaching." The leg pain, he attributes
to normal "growing pains." "All children get them," he assures you. Fast-
forward: It is one year and dozens of doctors later. Your daughter is still in
pain. In fact, the pain is much worse and has traveled to other areas of her
body. She is attending school sporadically, and she shows little interest in
the things she once loved, such as her friends and gymnastics. What's
more, you are still no closer to knowing what is causing the pain. Your
nerves are frazzled; you are missing work, are fighting with your husband,
and feel guilty all the time. "How did this happen?" you ask yourself.

Pain is much more than an uncomfortable sensation that we all
would like to keep our children from experiencing. It can affect a child's
ability to breathe easily, perform everyday tasks and activities, and eat
normally. It also interferes with sleep and energy, and it alters mood and
disrupts relationships.

You may be just beginning the journey to understanding your
child's pain, or you may have been struggling with it for years. You may
be feeling many of the symptoms of what I call the "parent pain burnout
syndrome"—fear, confusion, frustration, anger, and helplessness. You are
not alone. One in five children in the United States suffers from some
form of chronic pain. That means that at least the same number or more
parents are suffering right along with those children.

Pain, in one form or another, is a part of every child's life experience. Some children are fortunate to experience only common cuts and
bruises, whereas others experience more serious injury, illness, or disease.
Some types of pain can be useful, because they teach children what is dan-

gerous (e.g., touching a hot stove) or alert parents to a condition that needs immediate attention (e.g., acute pain in the right lower belly associated with appendicitis). However, chronic pain never serves a useful purpose. It is the most misunderstood of all childhood conditions for which parents seek pediatric help.

CHRONIC VERSUS ACUTE PAIN

Teresa, nine years old, had the flu and developed abdominal pain. Two different doctors told her that it was just the flu and not to worry. However, her belly pain got worse. It turned out that she had a ruptured appendix; she spent two weeks in the hospital. (Parents: Most cases of appendicitis are readily diagnosed not only by belly pain but also by physical examination and the child's white blood cell count, so please don't worry every time your child has a stomachache.)

Teresa had a five-inch incision from her navel to her pelvic bone that had to remain open to allow the wound to drain. She experienced severe postoperative and daily procedural pain when the surgeons cleaned her wound. After Teresa came home from the hospital, her mother, Deana, had to clean the wound so that it would continue to drain. This daily process caused Teresa excruciating pain. For Deana, performing this task while her child screamed in pain was torture. The wound eventually drained and healed, but Teresa's belly pain persisted.

Teresa started to fear going to the bathroom because of the pain and began having trouble sleeping at night. The director of pediatric surgery at the hospital and two specialists told Deana that Teresa's pain was "all in her head" and that she "was going to have to live with it." They also believed that Teresa must have "a low pain tolerance"—rather ironic, considering what she had already endured.

Finally, a gastroenterologist was consulted. He was appalled and told Deana, "No child should have to experience or live with this kind of pain." A simple statement, but it was a tremendous relief to both Teresa and her mom because they had begun to feel that they were crazy. Despite his empathy, however, the gastroenterologist did not know how to help Teresa.

Today, nearly five years later, Teresa still suffers from some pain, although she has found many ways to alleviate much of it—including massage, Iyengar yoga, biofeedback, and low doses of the antidepressant Elavil and the antianxiety drug Effexor.

* * *

Pain generally has two basic forms—acute and chronic. Although most people think of all pain as pretty much the same and so approach it the same way, there are important differences between the two. Approaching them with the same mind-set may result in prolonging a child's chronic pain. Also, inadequate treatment of acute pain or pain associated with medical procedures or injuries may actually worsen chronic pain or lead to the development of chronic pain.

Acute pain is usually a signal that there is some tissue injury, inflammation, or infection that may need immediate attention. For example, if your child burns his hand, he feels pain and withdraws it from the source of the burn. Thus, acute pain serves as a warning signal to take action. This is what we often refer to as pain that serves a purpose. Acute pain is typically brief and usually ends after the injury heals, the inflammation has subsided, or the stretch, contraction, or impingement on the body part has resolved. Examples of acute pain include the pain of a broken arm, postsurgical pain, acute gastroenteritis, menstrual cramps, a sore throat, pain from an ear infection, or muscle cramps from exercising more than you are used to. This type of pain can be mild to severe, but most acute pain conditions are readily diagnosable, which means that the source is fairly easily discovered.

Chronic pain, on the other hand, may or may not be symptomatic of underlying, ongoing tissue damage or chronic disease. It can persist long after the initial injury has healed (typically longer than three months) and no longer serves a useful warning function. Or it may have an ongoing cause, such as arthritis, cancer, nerve damage, or chronic infection. Chronic pain can hinder the body's ability to heal itself, and so the pain itself becomes the chronic problem.

Even with acute pain, physical movement, emotions, beliefs, and environmental factors (e.g., what doctors, nurses, and parents do and say) can affect the amount of pain a child experiences and even how long the pain lasts. With chronic pain, there is more opportunity for these factors to affect the pain as well as the child's ability to function—attend school, participate in athletics, and engage in social interaction. (I discuss these factors in detail in Chapter 5, "Factors That Contribute to Chronic Pain.") For these reasons, even pain related initially to known likely causes, like arthritis or surgery, can become more severe and continuous than would otherwise be expected.

Children who develop chronic pain are not pretending to have pain, even if it seems there is no reason for it. They are having real, honest-to-goodness pain and are suffering. Discovering the root of the problem and treating it sometimes means that doctors and parents must engage in detective work, which involves understanding all the different factors that are maintaining and increasing the pain and suffering. For most types of acute pain, such efforts are not typically needed.

Conventional treatments usually work for acute pain. For example, ibruprofen can reduce pain and inflammation for muscle aches, whereas morphine can be very effective for postsurgical pain. However, if acute pain is not well treated, the body's pain systems can become sensitized (turned on), and thus acute pain can lead to chronic pain. Furthermore, the traditional medical model, with its emphasis on the doctor being responsible for "curing" patients, as well as its reliance on procedures such as surgeries or nerve blocks and on pain medications, is often ineffective for ameliorating chronic pain, especially in children. And because there has been little research on treatments for chronic pain until recently, one of three things happens: Children are subjected to unnecessary surgical procedures and drugs, they go without adequate treatment, or their complaints are completely discounted.

Although I have seen many children with chronic pain who have been undertreated, I also get patients who have undergone unnecessary surgical procedures or are prescribed potent drugs simply because their doctor has run out of ideas and feels pressure to do something to alleviate the child's suffering. Many of my colleagues tell me that the pressure to do something often comes from well-meaning parents who can't bear to see their child suffer anymore.

Unfortunately, in most cases, the surgery does little to stem the pain, and in many cases, makes it worse. And not only do opioids (such as morphine) not help many types of pain (other than to reduce some anxiety or put the child to sleep) but they can actually prolong the pain by decreasing the production of one of the body's key pain-fighting chemicals (neurotransmitters called enkephalins and endorphins). These chemicals are similar in structure to opioids, and if the child is getting opioids from elsewhere (not made by the body), the factory in the body where these chemicals are produced decreases production. This means that the body's natural pain-control system begins to work less and less effectively, keeping the pain cycle going.

The fact is most physicians are not as adequately trained in dealing with chronic pain as they are in treating acute pain. I want to help you to understand what chronic pain is, how to identify it, and what factors can contribute to the pain, keep it going, or actually increase it. In the pages to follow, I provide some basic lessons about pain.

THE ABCS OF PAIN

Lesson 1: Pain Perception Is Regulated by the Brain

When your child feels pain—for example, when she bruises her knee—the pain is really a reaction to signals transmitted throughout her body, sent via sensory nerves from the pain source (in this case, the knee), through nerve fibers in the back part of the spinal cord, to her brain, where she perceives them as pain. Thus you need a brain to feel pain. Stopping the nerve signals from reaching parts of the brain that receive these signals is the reason anesthesia was developed.

However, during surgery there are still pain signals being carried by sensory nerves from the surgical site, up the spinal cord, and into the brain. That's why the anesthesiologist will also administer your child medicines (opioid analgesics) to reduce the pain signals so that when she wakes up after the anesthesia wears off, she will not suddenly have a barrage of pain signals reaching her brain all at once. Additional opioids also are given during the healing postoperative period until the pain signals are reduced.

Chronic pain develops when the area of the brain that has been receiving pain signals becomes activated and remains active even if there are no more pain signals stimulating it. These activated pain perception areas in the brain can continue on automatic pilot. An extreme example of this process at work is phantom limb pain, or pain in an arm or leg that has been amputated. The pain continues in the limb even though it has been removed because the brain is still registering the pain signals that the painful limb was sending to the brain before the amputation. Even after the limb is amputated, that part of the brain has been turned on and keeps reading pain. Almost all people who have a limb amputated feel phantom sensations such as touch, movement, and change in temperature for about a year or so. However, if these individuals had pain in the limb before the amputation, they are more likely to have phantom limb pain, because the primary signal in that area of the brain before the amputation was pain rather than another sensation.

Doctors therefore work hard to reduce pain. The best ways to treat phantom limb pain are approaches such as hypnosis that work directly on the pain perception areas of the brain, rather than methods aimed at the remaining part of the limb.

When I first came to UCLA, I was asked to consult on the case of a 16-year-old boy who had a bone tumor at the base of his femur and had had the leg amputated above the knee. Gary had been suffering with leg pain for quite a while before he came to UCLA and the tumor was diagnosed. Despite a successful surgery, he could not function because of what he described as "squeezing, burning pain." He had been treated with large doses of opioids, which helped only when they put him totally to sleep. I first tried medications to address the pain related to nerve signaling problems. These helped a little, but he was still suffering. I began helping him use his imagination to disrupt the pain signals that had remained on automatic pilot even though his limb, and thus the original cause of the pain, had been amputated.

At that time, less was known about the biology of pain perception than is known today. I saw Gary weekly, and he developed his own set of mental images that typically involved playing soccer. (He had been a star soccer player before his bone tumor.) While he played soccer in his mind, the pain was gone and he could feel himself running on the field. Over time, the pain diminished—even during the nonimagery time—until he noticed that the pain didn't bother him anymore and he was finally able to begin physical rehabilitation with a prosthetic leg.

Since that time, scientists have learned more about the areas of the brain where pain perception takes place. There are different areas of the brain that control pain sensation (what it feels like and where it is coming from) and pain suffering (how distressing it is). Research with modern imaging techniques such as positron emission tomography (PET) scanning and functional magnetic resonance imaging (f MRI) have shown that even suggestions of sensations (as is done during hypnosis and imagery therapy) can affect one part of the brain perception areas and not another.

Lesson 2: Pain Is Physical and Psychological

All pain is both physical (sensory) and psychological (emotional). As discussed above, it is the brain—not the point of injury or even where the pain is felt—that registers the sensation and emotional suffering of pain. We all have emotional reactions to pain. Emotions and beliefs can directly affect nerve signaling and neurotransmitters that underlie the physiology of pain. In fact, in the experience of pain there is no way to separate the parts of the pain that relate to its underlying biology and those that relate to emotions such as anxiety, sadness, or fear.

René Descartes (1596–1650), one of the most important Western philosophers of the past few centuries, believed that the mind and body were two distinct entities. This led him to argue that there was a one-to-one correlation between the pain stimulus and the amount of pain experienced. That is, if you touched something hot (the stimulus), the pain would travel from your finger to your brain and register pain. In principle, this is only partially correct. The pain signal would indeed reach the brain. However, according to this theory, each person would experience the same amount of pain from the same amount of pain stimulus, and we know that this isn't true. What Descartes didn't realize was that the mind and body are intimately connected.

Neural networks (nerve signals) and areas of the brain are active when we think and feel emotions. Through the biological processes of thinking and feeling, we can either increase pain by worrying about it and believing that it will get worse or decrease pain by keeping our mind on other things and believing that it will get better.

When we think and feel, there are changes in our brain's neurotransmitters (chemicals). Depending on what we are thinking or feeling, we may also have changes in stress hormones, blood flow, and other physiological activities in our body. For example, think of the last time you felt scared. Did you notice that your heart began to race, your hands became sweaty, and your breathing sped up? We now have the tools like fMRI and other techniques to see what areas of the brain are active when we are laughing, depressed, excited, or in pain. These areas communicate with one another and can influence each other. This is why all pain is both biological and psychological.

Lesson 3: How Feelings and Thoughts Increase or Decrease Pain

Pain signals begin at nociceptors (special small nerve fibers that carry pain or negative sensory messages) and travel as nerve impulses upward through the spinal cord and into the brain, both of which compose the central nervous system (CNS). Neurotransmitters carry the signals from one nerve fiber to another and to different centers in the brain. Depending on whether there is stress, anxiety, depression, or even anger, the original pain signals can be amplified or increased as they progress up to the brain.

This means that feelings and thoughts can actually increase the volume of the pain signals, like turning up the sound on the TV. Similarly, reducing anxiety can turn down the volume on the pain signaling. When we feel anxious, our sympathetic nervous system (SNS) becomes active. This causes our heart to speed up and other physical symptoms to occur. Anxiety increases our pain experience by increasing the pain signals and by increasing activity in the pain perception areas of the brain, especially the part of our brain that perceives the distress related to pain.

Beliefs and thoughts also can impact pain. Try to think of a time when you injured yourself, had a headache, or, if you're a woman, had menstrual cramps. When you focused your attention on the pain, it got worse. This is because you cleared your brain of other things, leaving lots of room for pain signals. If you then worried that the pain was a sign of something serious or that it was going to get worse, the pain probably did get worse. This is because the belief that the pain meant something serious made you worry. As you started to worry, the chemicals in your brain began to change, and those changes increased the pain signals.

Now remember a time when you were in pain but were distracted by something. The pain moved from foreground into background while you focused on other things, and the same pain bothered you less. If you are in pain and worried about it, even just telling yourself that it will be fine and that you will get through it can lessen the pain by reducing the stress chemicals in the brain and nervous system as you begin to relax.

Lesson 4: Memories Can Affect Pain

Other factors, such as past memories of pain, may play a role in the sensory feeling of the pain (how strong it is, for example) and the suffering component (how much it bothers you). With each pain experience, memory circuits for that pain experience can be created and recalled at a future time. Which pain experiences get stored depends on how your child is feeling at the time he experiences the pain.

If a child has a significant pain experience (such as with an injury or surgery) and is also stressed while he is in pain, his body will become more sensitive to pain. Anxiety appears to increase the relationship between pain and memory of pain; that is, it helps lay down the memory of pain so it can be recalled more easily later. This can serve a protective function in the short term but can be harmful if the stress continues.

For example, if you are injured in an automobile accident, the acute stress (shock) of the accident might cause you not to feel the pain at the time of the accident. This is called stress-induced analgesia. This phenomenon was also noted during World War II when soldiers on the battlefield had arms blown off and didn't feel the pain until they were safe in the medical unit. Acute intense stress can block pain signals, but as the stress is reduced, that stressful and painful experience is more likely to be laid down in memory, especially if there is pain with the stress and the pain is not well treated. Later, if the brain is activated with worries or fear, those pain memories can be retrieved and the pain can be felt or experienced again. (For more on memory and chronic pain, see Chapter 5, "Factors That Contribute to Chronic Pain.")

Lesson 5: The Body Has a Natural Pain Control System

Fortunately, we all have a natural pain-control system in our body that acts to block, reduce, or change pain, striking a balance between pain transmission and control. I like to think of the pain system as a radio or TV, with you as the regulator of the volume. If someone or something comes along and turns up the volume so that it is too loud (too much pain), you'll want to turn down the volume until you have the sound just right (normal sensation, but no pain).

The goal of pain treatment is to get the body's internal volume system to work properly, as it did before the pain began. You want to be able to feel normal acute pain, as in injuries or inflammation, so that you can take action to prevent further injury. However, you want your body's pain-control system to regulate the pain signals (the volume) so that the system is not always on high volume, leaving you in a lot of pain.

You don't need chronic pain. It takes a toll on your body. Another way of thinking about chronic pain is to imagine never getting a tune-up for your car. After a while, it still runs, but it becomes less and less efficient, burning more oil, using more gas, damaging the engine, until it finally stops running. Treatment for chronic pain is similar to a tune-up. Your pain system isn't broken, but it needs adjusting so that it can run well again.

Lesson 6: Pain Can Be Controlled

If your child's natural pain-control system isn't functioning properly, the pain can be controlled by preventing the pain signals from reaching the brain or reducing or blocking them anywhere along the pathway from the frame of the body (skin, muscles, bone), internal organs, autonomic nervous system (ANS), spinal cord, or in the brain itself. This can be achieved by using medication or nondrug treatments to block or reduce the pain.

If the pain signals never reach the brain or are altered inside the brain, either your child won't feel the pain or it won't bother him anymore. Remember, there are two areas in the brain for pain perception: (1) pain perception for bother/distress/suffering and (2) pain perception for pain sensation (where it is located and what it feels like). In treatment, the most important area to target first is the area related to pain suffering. This is because if your child feels the pain but it no longer bothers him as much as before, he can begin to function and do more, like go to school or play with friends. The more he can function, even with pain, the more quickly the pain will go away or be reduced.

Opioids (narcotics such as morphine) work by reducing the activity in the pain perception area for suffering. If you've ever taken an opioid such as Vicodin after having a dental procedure or surgery, you may remember that you still felt the pain but weren't bothered by it. You may have even smiled while you talked about your pain (sometimes called the "opioid grin").

I believe that the best and longest-lasting treatments are those that help the body's pain-control system to work optimally. Medications such as Tylenol with codeine or Vicodin can reduce pain in some situations but do nothing to help the body's natural pain-control system work efficiently. In fact, opioids block the body's own natural endorphin production, an important part of the pain-control system, which can actually result in more pain.

Medications such as selective serotonin reuptake inhibitors (SSRIs, or antidepressants) or tricyclic antidepressants that increase the body's levels of the neurotransmitters serotonin and norepinephrine, respectively, are far preferable to analgesics (painkillers). (Serotonin and norepinephrine are important neurotransmitters involved in the body's pain-control system.) There are many nondrug therapies such as acupuncture and massage that can influence these natural neurotransmittors. Also, there are lots of nondrug treatments (e.g., biofeedback, yoga, hypnotherapy) that can directly alter the brain's pain perception area for suffering. (I discuss these treatments in Chapter 8, "Complementary and Alternative Therapies.")

Lesson 7: Different Kinds of Pain React to Different Treatments
The origin of some pain is neuropathic, whereas other pain is nociceptive. Neuropathic pain is caused by injury or damage to nerve tissue or by disordered nerve signaling without actual physical nerve damage or inflammation. This kind of pain is often felt as a burning or stabbing pain and typically is located in one part of the body. Examples of neuropathic pain include sciatica or the pain of a pinched nerve or pain associated with shingles or CRPS type I (formerly known as RSD), in which the skin and underlying tissue in the affected body part often feels supersensitive and hurts.

Nociceptive pain is caused by an injury, inflammation, disease, or stress on certain tissues such as in muscle spasms. Such pain is experienced by a child as an ongoing dull ache or pressure if the source of the pain is solid organs such as the liver, spleen, kidneys, muscle, bone covering, or other tissues. If the child complains of cramping, the source of the pain may be hollow organs such as intestines, bladder, uterus, or fallopian tubes. Examples of nociceptive pain include arthritis pain, gastroenteritis pain, menstrual cramps, or tension headaches.

However, a child with chronic pain may have pain that starts as nociceptive pain (if the problem begins with infection, injury, or inflammation) and then becomes neuropathic—after the initial problem resolves, the nervous system keeps misfiring. For example, a common way for IBS to start is with an episode of acute gastroenteritis. Typically, a viral infection in the intestinal tract causes inflammation, with intestinal cramping and often diarrhea, nausea, vomiting, and perhaps fever. In some children, the inflammation goes away but the pain remains: The inflammation sets off the pain signals, but after the infection clears, the pain signals between the brain and the intestines go on automatic pilot and keep firing.

Sometimes children experience mixed pain, or a combination of neuropathic and nociceptive pain. They may have an ongoing case of nociceptive pain, as in arthritis, for example. However, if the pain continues and isn't addressed, the CNS and certain areas of the brain can become hypersensitized and turned on. This increase in the volume of the entire pain transmission system can cause the pain to be severe and more than it might have been with just the arthritis alone.

It is important to differentiate between the types of pain, because treatments may differ depending on the types of and reasons for the pain. If inflammation is the cause of the pain (e.g., ulcerative colitis or Crohn's disease in the intestinal tract, called inflammatory bowel disease, or IBD), then we need to treat the inflammation to treat the pain. This type of treatment will be different from that used, for example, in IBS, where there no longer is any inflammation, even if the pain started with inflammation.

PAIN IS NOT IMAGINED—IT IS REAL

Ten-year-old Jane suffered with severe knee pain. Four doctors had already been unsuccessful in treating her, and the pain in her right knee had steadily progressed to the point where she was unable to straighten it. Jane said that the pain made her limp until she could no longer walk and that it felt like "something was not right inside." After a misdiagnosis by the pediatrician, she saw an orthopedist who said that MRI showed torn cartilage (although Jane did not remember injuring herself). Jane had surgery to repair the cartilage. But the pain was worse after surgery. She described with tears the "torture" that she experienced with physical therapy. Jane was referred to a rheumatologist, who gave her steroids and knee injections. Jane's mother said that after no improvement and normal tests, the rheumatologist told Jane, "Enough pillows. Straighten your legs . . . I have other patients with real pain. . . . If you don't start moving your leg, I'll put it in a brace and crank it up at night!" She said that Jane cried throughout that visit and refused to return.

• • •

One of the issues that can complicate the diagnosis and treatment of chronic pain in children is that nagging question, "Is the pain real or imagined?" Though this question comes up in the treatment of pain in adults, it is much more frequently on the minds of physicians and parents when it comes to children's complaints about pain, because children are often considered to be less reliable than adults in reporting symptoms and degrees of pain they experience.

I believe that if a child complains of pain, the pain is real and the child is suffering. The job of parents and physicians is to figure out what might have started the pain and, more importantly, what is keeping the pain going. Typically the pain is continuing not because of one single thing such as torn cartilage but more commonly from an array of factors. Jane's frustration and anxiety over not being believed only served to increase her pain. She was pushed to move her knee before she learned how to do that successfully and cope with the pain so that it wouldn't bother her so much.

In diagnosing the cause of pain, typically doctors first think about all of the disease-related possible causes. They conduct tests or procedures to look for pathological evidence (e.g., evidence of inflammation, a bacteria, tissue injury, or mechanical obstruction). If the test results are negative for any identifiable disease, they may say that the cause of the pain is likely "functional." This means that the nerve signals have become functionally impaired. Your child's doctor may also use the word *psycho-*

somatic, meaning that the pain is "psychological" in origin. Many parents, children, and even some doctors think that this means that the pain is not "real" (that is, having no biological basis), and often the child is referred to a mental health professional. However, we now know that there is a biological and neurochemical process that leads to the types of pain that are often called functional or psychosomatic.

Dr. Allen Finley, medical director of Pediatric Pain Management at the IWK Health Centre in Halifax, Nova Scotia, offers this advice to children whose family, friends, or doctors don't understand or believe they are in pain: "We tell patients, 'You know more about your pain than anyone else. You should think of these people as just needing to be educated, and you are the expert.'"

All pain is caused by a complex interaction between the brain and the rest of the body. Just because doctors cannot find the cause of the pain does not mean it is purely psychological. IBS is called a functional bowel disorder by gastroenterologists. We don't know exactly how IBS happens or why it happens to some children. There may be genetic reasons (there is a higher incidence in twins than in nontwin siblings), familial reasons (there is an even higher likelihood of a twin's having IBS if a parent has IBS than if the other twin has IBS), stress-related reasons, and others. The bottom line is that in functional pain, the pain-signaling system is not working normally. In most such cases, results of any test done to find a disease or illness will come back negative.

The goal of treatment is to turn on the body's natural pain-control system so it can work properly again.

CHILDREN ARE OFTEN
UNDERTREATED FOR PAIN

Despite advances in pediatric pain medicine, children are still frequently undertreated for pain, especially acute pain, such as postsurgical pain, trauma, and medical procedure pain. There are a variety of possible reasons for this: misunderstanding or underestimating the incidence or seriousness of pediatric pain and its consequences, individual and cultural attitudes about pain, the complexities and effort involved in assessing pain in children, inadequate education, and insufficient research in pediatric pain. Furthermore, some physicians and parents are hesitant to use common pain medications to treat children with acute pain for fear these medications are too strong and that the child might either be harmed or become addicted.

There are a few important points to remember:

- First, if your child says that she is in pain, she is. In my opinion, expressing the attitude that "the pain is all in your head" should be avoided at all costs. Such a limited way of thinking can lead to unnecessary tests, procedures, and medical treatments or, conversely, to a lack of empathy that may result in substandard care for your child. Ultimately, and most important, it may undermine the child's confidence in his ability to get better.

- Second, your job, together with your child's primary care physician, is to understand what factors are contributing to your child's experience of pain—that is, what has caused the pain to become chronic, what is increasing his suffering, and what is maintaining the pain.

- Third, learn how to address these factors—not simply by using an analgesic to reduce the pain itself, as you would for an acute pain problem such as an injury or a sore throat. As with any disease, there can be emotional, cognitive, and environmental contributors to the pain, adding in varying degrees to the overall problem.

Understanding the general principles of pain (how it is created, continued, or turned off) allows you to help your child cope better with the pain, and you will be more successful at finding a physician who has some understanding of current pediatric pain treatment. Adult-oriented pain programs typically do not have physicians with specific pediatric pain management training, and treating children in pain is very different from treating adults. For example, invasive procedures such as epidural and other nerve blocks are used far less often in children than in adults, and nondrug therapies are used more often in children. Also, drugs used for pain in adults may not be appropriate for children. As pediatric pain research continues, general pediatricians and family medicine physicians are becoming more knowledgeable and would be the first physician to go to for help with your child in pain. I strongly urge you to see your child's primary care physician first before you seek specialty help.

{ CHAPTER TWO }

Diseases and Illnesses Associated with Chronic Pain

Disease is cured by the body itself, not by doctors or remedies.
—JOHN HARVEY KELLOGG, M.D.

Damian is a 15-year-old young man with sickle cell disease, an inherited genetic disease. Over the years, Damian had experienced bouts of pain in his chest, stomach, arms, and legs caused by the blockage of blood flow due to the sickled shape of his blood cells.

In the past, Damian's sickle cell pain "crises," as he called them, had occurred as infrequently as once a year, but from age 13 to age 15 he had been having them more often and was increasingly visiting the local emergency room (ER) and being hospitalized for his pain. Sometimes the pain was brief; other times it lasted hours, days, or even weeks. He had begun to tire more easily and was having problems fighting infections. He tried his best to manage his pain at home so that he did not need to go to the ER or be admitted to the hospital, but it was becoming difficult.

Damian always tried to maintain a sense of humor about his pain and was often upbeat and joking with his doctors and the nurses who treated him. But in the last two to three years, his mood had changed. He became sullen. The doctors began to wonder if Damian was coming to the hospital "just to get drugs," and Damian became suspicious and did not trust the doctors. His more intense and frequent pain crises forced him to rely more and more on the ER and the hospital for intravenous (IV) fluids and stronger pain medications.

• • •

In this chapter, I review some diseases that are or can be associated with chronic pain: sickle cell disease, arthritis, and IBD. The amount and frequency of pain in a child with any of these diseases can vary. Some children have very little pain, whereas others have significant pain. The differences relate to whether there are other factors present such as anxiety, learning disabilities, and coping issues that are increasing or decreasing the pain signals.

For example, for most children with arthritis, chronic pain is not a huge issue, if the arthritis is well managed. But chronic pain can become a problem if the child is anxious or stressed or has had physical or emotional trauma. Normal, or expected, pain from an illness or disease becomes chronic when the body's sensory nerves become hypersensitive and bombard the brain with pain signals. The body gets overloaded, the normal pain-control mechanisms don't work well, and the child develops a pain disorder that will not go away by simply "fixing" the disease.

You can see how this works in the cases that follow. In each case, the child's disease typically could be easily controlled with medication, but is not because the child's nervous system is not working properly. In each case, chronic pain develops. (For a detailed discussion of the factors related to chronic pain, see Chapter 5, "Factors That Contribute to Chronic Pain.")

SICKLE CELL DISEASE

Sickle cell disease (SCD) is an inherited blood disorder that causes chronic destruction of red blood cells, episodes of intense pain, vulnerability to infections, organ damage, and, in some cases, early death. It is most prevalent among African-Americans and Hispanic-Americans. Health experts estimate that 1 of every 500 African-American children and 1 of every 1,400 Hispanic-American children are born with SCD.

People with SCD have red blood cells that contain an abnormal type of hemoglobin (the oxygen-carrying part of the red blood cells). Sometimes these red blood cells become sickled (crescent shaped) and have difficulty passing through small blood vessels. When sickle-shaped cells block small blood vessels, less blood can reach that part of the body. Tissue that does not receive a normal blood flow eventually becomes damaged.

If organs or body parts are deprived of oxygen, there is a buildup of certain substances at nerve endings, and pain signals are activated. Imagine your arm is being squeezed by a blood pressure cuff that keeps getting tighter and tighter until your arm turns blue. After a while, your arm will begin to ache and the pain may become unbearable. This is often the type of pain experienced by children and adolescents with SCD.

Children and adolescents with SCD can also develop headaches and low back pain from chronic muscle spasm and lack of oxygen in their spine. They can experience joint pain, especially in the hip, when the head of the femur (the large bone in the thigh) at the hip is destroyed from a lack of blood and oxygen. This hip condition also can cause a deep, aching referred pain—pain coming from one part of the body that is felt in another part—in the lower thigh above the knee.

We do not know if there is something endemic to SCD that causes some children to have frequent, repetitive bouts of pain and others to have a milder, intermittent form. What we do know is that the pain can vary wildly depending on the child.

Most of the time, sickle cell pain crises can be prevented with regular hydration (drinking lots of liquids), exercise, and a healthy diet and by preventing exposure to low-oxygen situations such as mountain-climbing. However, for some people with SCD, even these steps do not prevent pain. Management of a pain crisis begins with having a treatment plan and medication set up in advance of pain onset.

A Child with Sickle Cell Disease

I first met Damian when he was 13 years old. When he was younger than 11 or 12, he rarely came to the hospital. According to those who knew him, he was a happy boy who did well in school, had friends, and liked to ride his bike in the neighborhood with his brothers. However, as he entered adolescence, several things happened. In middle school, he found it difficult to keep up, especially in math, and he received poor, close to failing, grades. He also had a very traumatic personal experience around this time.

In retrospect, although no one knew it at the time, Damian probably had a learning disability (most likely in math), and by the time he entered middle school he was having an increasingly difficult time, as the schoolwork became more complex and plentiful compared to elementary school.

By the time I met him, Damian had become introverted and talked little about his personal life or feelings. The best I could do was to treat his immediate pain during the sickle cell pain crises. It wasn't until Damian was 15 that he began to trust me enough to talk about his family life. Finally, I understood some of the reasons that his pain had been getting worse and that he was finding it more difficult to cope with his pain than he had when he was younger.

When Damian was 13, his older brother, whom he adored and

looked up to, became involved in a gang and was killed in a gang-related shooting. Damian, who was standing next to his brother at the time, witnessed the shooting. According to Damian, a car drove by, he heard gunfire, and the next thing he saw was his brother lying on the ground with blood "pouring out of his chest." His brother looked up at him and then died before the ambulance arrived.

Shortly after the incident, Damian became withdrawn and kept to himself. He became fearful and seemed always on alert. He developed trouble sleeping, not only when he was in pain. He became more fatigued during the day. He had increased trouble concentrating in school and began to fall further behind in his classes.

He would tell me later that he blamed himself for his brother's death because his brother had come home to help Damian fix his bike, and they were walking to the store to get some parts that they needed when the shooting occurred. Damian was certain that if he hadn't called his brother to come home and help him, his brother would be alive today.

One of the results of SCD is stunted height. Because of a lack of circulation and oxygen to the spinal bones, they collapse on one another and the spine shortens. During adolescence, as other boys his age were going through growth spurts related to puberty, Damian remained short. Some bullies at school began to tease him about being short. He was very insecure about his size and looked for other ways to feel big. He began to smoke, stay up late, and skip school. His parents, still distraught over the death of their older son, did not know how to help Damian. They warned him that he was going to become a gang member and be killed like his brother if he didn't start going to school and doing his homework. Damian and his parents, who had always been quite close, became alienated from one another. Although Damian and his parents were all suffering from the loss of brother/son, they were unable to talk about their grief or provide comfort to one another. This is a common response in families who have suffered a traumatic loss.

Damian's performance in school plummeted further after his brother's death, and the sickle cell pain crises increased in frequency and intensity. He often skipped his doctor appointments and did not take care of himself as he once had in order to keep the pain in check; he stopped taking his medications and refused to let his parents help him. Damian often ended up in the ER, writhing in pain. Typically, by the time a doctor saw him, he was in such pain that he would be screaming for "a morphine shot." Often, he was not given enough medication and would ask for more.

The doctors became suspicious that Damian was using the hospital ER to get drugs. They thought that they were helping him by reducing the doses and delaying the morphine injections. The nurses would talk among themselves about Damian's "drug-seeking behavior." They determined that it was suspicious that he seemed perfectly comfortable watching TV or playing video games in his hospital bed one minute and then, when he was asked to rate his pain only minutes later, he would rate it a 10 on a scale of 0 to 10, where 10 is the worst pain. It just wasn't possible, they argued.

What had happened to this once close-knit family and happy boy with a wonderful grin and great sense of humor? Just a few years earlier, he and his family had easily been able to manage his pain at home with little disruption to their daily lives. Now he had become a withdrawn, sullen, mistrustful, "drug-seeking" teenager who was in constant pain and disconnected from his peers, family, and the doctors who were trying to help him. What was affecting his pain experience?

Beliefs and emotions can play an important role in biological pain signaling and in the personal experience of pain and suffering. This is true for children with all types of diseases. For Damian, the day of his brother's death began a downward spiral in his condition. He relived the incident over and over again in his mind.

Damian was suffering from classical symptoms of post-traumatic stress disorder (PTSD): difficulty sleeping, flashbacks of the traumatic event, difficulty concentrating, feeling always on alert and startling more easily, seeming to be emotionally detached, and avoiding activities or places associated with the traumatic event. Though Damian's story is dramatic, there are more subtle traumas that can cause PTSD. For example, a car accident (even if no one was seriously hurt), a sports accident, or witnessing or learning about the death of a classmate can each cause PTSD symptoms, which, in turn, can worsen pain. PTSD can also be caused by overzealous and invasive medical procedures in the search for the cause of a chronic pain problem.

In PTSD, the nervous system changes at a biological level in its response to stress. This happened for Damian. He startled more easily and his body became hyperreactive to emotional and physical stressors. This increase in the arousal or turn-on of his sympathetic nervous system (SNS) (the part of his nervous system that reacts to stress) also affected his sensory nervous system (the part of his nervous system that carries pain signals to his brain). The SNS connects with (or talks to) the sensory nervous system in a way that increases the volume or magnitude of pain signals to the brain and thus increases pain. For someone with SCD, being chronically stressed and having symptoms of PTSD with a turned-on SNS can be particularly problematic. One of the hormones that circulates in the body with a turned-on SNS is adrenaline. Not only does adrenaline cause the typical symptoms that you feel when you are anxious—for example, your heart races and your hands sweat—but it also can cause blood vessels to narrow or constrict. For someone with SCD, narrowed blood vessels can cause more sickled cells to block vessels, resulting in much more pain.

Damian's pain crises were becoming more frequent, more distressing, and he was unable to see an end to the pain. He saw his life "going down the tubes." Because Damian was suffering from PTSD symptoms, he also shut down emotionally and he seemed to have an "I don't care" attitude about his medical condition and health in general. At the time, Damian was also entering adolescence, which brought other stressors, such as his need for and confusion over independence, and social and sexual experimentation.

I use Damian's story as an example of some of the factors that can contribute to a child's chronic pain experience. Some of these factors are developmental, such as a child entering adolescence (typically at age 11 or 12 years); some are cognitive, such as a previously unsuspected learning disability; and some are emotional, such as an acute major trauma leading to PTSD, or new stressors from school, home, or peers. Even subtle life changes such as a move to a different neighborhood, a change in schools, or the beginning of the school year can cause pain to grow worse. (For a further discussion of the role of changes, stress, and other factors that contribute to pain, see Chapter 5, "Factors That Contribute to Chronic Pain.")

SCD is associated with recurrent bouts of pain, as are a number of other diseases. However, pain is not inevitable, even from these diseases. There are reasons for the pain, and the pain can be prevented or at least managed. What you will discover is that even though diseases may differ and reasons for increased pain can be varied, there are some common ways to treat any type of pain.

INFLAMMATORY BOWEL DISEASE

IBD is a condition of ongoing or recurrent inflammation in the intestinal tract. (IBD is not to be confused with irritable bowel syndrome, or IBS, which I discuss in Chapter 3, "Chronic Pain Conditions," on pages 70–77.) There are several forms of IBD. Ulcerative colitis is an IBD that is limited to the colon (large intestine). Early signs include left-sided abdominal pain that improves after bowel movements, joint pain, and progressive loosening of the stools, which are often bloody. Severe abdominal pain and bloody stools can create disabling symptoms for children when the disease is first diagnosed or during times of increased inflammation. Treatment is aimed at reducing inflammation in the colon, usually by specific anti-inflammatory medication. Removal of the colon is an option of last resort.

Crohn's disease is another type of IBD in which there can be patchy inflammation that can involve all the layers of the wall of the intestine. The early signs of Crohn's disease in children are often vague, making diagnosis difficult. Abdominal pain over the navel or on the right side is most common and may appear long before pervasive diarrhea. There also may be joint pain and fever before there are any changes in bowel patterns. Decreased appetite and weight loss are often symptoms misdiagnosed as anorexia nervosa, school anxiety, or other psychological problems.

There are effective anti-inflammatory treatments that can prevent or get rid of the inflammation, and this usually resolves the pain. Not every child with IBD actually has abdominal pain, even though there may be small areas of intestinal inflammation. However, in some children who might be at risk for the development of chronic pain (those who have an anxiety disorder, PTSD, or other condition associated with a hypersensitive nervous system), severe bouts of inflammatory-related abdominal pain or surgery can set off what is called phantom intestinal pain. In this case, the nerves carrying pain signals from the intestines to the brain get turned on and the signals become magnified so that the brain perceives just as much pain as if there were active inflammation, even though the intestines may be fine after anti-inflammatory treatment. It is called phantom pain because it can occur even if the colon has been removed.

There are sometimes outside-the-intestine manifestations of IBD, including arthritis or arthralgias (joint pain without inflammation) and skin rashes. However, the hallmark of IBD is inflammation of the intestine, usually with abdominal pain.

A Child with Inflammatory Bowel Disease

Fifteen-year-old Marcia's Crohn's disease was diagnosed when she was 13. She was treated with medications until all signs of inflammation were gone, as shown by endoscopy, colonoscopy, intestinal biopsies, and blood tests. Yet her abdominal pain continued, and she required multiple hospitalizations during which she was treated with IV opioids. Marcia was unable to attend school. Her gastroenterologist had tried treating her with newer experimental drugs for Crohn's disease, but her pain continued.

Marcia was referred to me for help with pain management. I learned that she attended a private school where she felt that most students were smarter than she. She said that she had been having trouble keeping up even before she began missing school. Marcia said that math was her most difficult subject and that she was in danger of failing. Her parents believed that she was gifted and wanted her to have the best education possible. They believed that she was just not trying hard enough.

I also learned that Marcia was a worrier. She worried about her parents' marriage, her health, her grades, and her friendships. She was beginning to feel isolated from her peer groups at school because of the amount of school that she had missed, and she believed that the cliques at school now excluded her. She had become demanding at home, and her parents were frustrated with her, saying that nothing they did pleased her.

Marcia focused much of our session on her pain and felt that it was unbearable and wanted some medication that would "take it away." Her parents were upset that the doctors could not "fix" their daughter.

I suspected that Marcia had a learning disability, which can become a major stressor if not addressed. Marcia underwent educational and neuropsychological testing and was found to have average intelligence (despite her parents' expectations that she was highly gifted), and she was far below the levels of most of the other students in her classes for gifted students. Feeling less able academically, Marcia had begun to feel "dumb." She also had missed so much school that she had fallen far behind.

Marcia's story illustrates several points. The first is that Marcia exhibited many symptoms of a generalized anxiety disorder. She worried intensely about many things, was always on alert, and had sleep problems. Though anxiety does not cause pain, it can worsen pain by increasing the volume of pain signals. Marcia's pain, her constant worry about her Crohn's disease, and her underlying anxiety disorder combined to create a sensory nervous system that was always turned on. Also, her belly became the constant focus of her attention, which only magnified the pain further. The more pain she had, the more she worried that she would develop more pain than she could tolerate. The problem was no longer in her intestines, but in her nerve signaling system and ultimately in her brain. The downward pain spiral had begun.

Marcia's treatment plan was aimed at several areas. The first order of business was to help her academically. Marcia was put in a more appropriate class where she felt smarter and could handle the workload. Additional tutoring was arranged so that she could catch up with the work she had missed. Marcia also was prescribed anti-inflammatory medication for the IBD and an antianxiety medication (an SSRI called Celexa) to reduce her anxiety enough to help her sleep. Last, she started cognitive-behavioral therapy (CBT).

CBT involves learning techniques to stop catastrophic thinking such as *The pain will get worse and I won't be able to handle it and I don't know what I am going to do*. Marcia was taught to take control of the thoughts by thinking instead, *I know what to do. . . . I can take some slow, deep breaths. . . . I know that I can handle this*. (For more on CBT, see Chapter 9, "Individual and Family Therapy," pages 190–192.) Finally, Marcia learned relaxation techniques such as breathing exercises and progressive muscle relaxation.

Gradually, Marcia was able to calm herself when she started to panic, a strategy that helped keep her nervous system in check, which eventually reduced her pain. Marcia was also encouraged to become more physically active. She started to walk for 30 minutes a day and took up Iyengar yoga, which made her feel more confident, which in turn helped her to engage in social and physical activities again. (For more on Iyengar yoga, see Chapter 8, "Complementary and Alternative Therapies," pages 167–171.) Marcia returned to a normal life. As she did so, her pain mostly resolved. Now the pain only occasionally flares up as part of her Crohn's disease, and without all the other stressors to exacerbate it, the pain is easily treated with medication.

JUVENILE ARTHRITIS

Often misunderstood as a disease of the elderly, arthritis can occur in anyone, without regard for age. It can bring intense pain to young adults, children, and even babies. Arthritis is an autoimmune disease that can invade every aspect of a child's life—physical, emotional, and social. More than 250,000 children in the United States have some form of arthritis. It can start as early as infancy and will last a lifetime. Juvenile arthritis is medically different from the adult form of rheumatoid or osteoarthritis and in many cases can be more severe. It can cause joint deformities and affect a child's skin, eyes, and internal organs.

Arthritis is an actual inflammation in the joints that causes the sensory nerve endings to transmit signals to the pain centers in the brain, resulting in joint pain. As I described earlier, pain signaling can be set off by many things, even minor injury where there is no tissue damage or inflammation. The pain can be of the same intensity with or without inflammation because the signals come from the same nerves. (The term *arthralgia* is used to indicate arthritis-like joint pain without noticeable inflammation, such as that experienced during the flu.)

There are different causes of childhood arthritis. The most common is called juvenile rheumatoid arthritis (JRA), an autoimmune condition involving primarily pain and inflammation in the joints. Sometimes only a single joint is involved (monoarticular arthritis), sometimes a few joints (pauciarticular arthritis) and sometimes many joints (polyarticular). In some cases, other parts of the body are involved, such as the eyes, where there may be inflammation of the uvea, the part of the eye that includes the iris. There are other, less common, causes of arthritis, besides JRA, such as arthritis associated with IBD, infections of the joints, and other autoimmune diseases such as systemic lupus erythematosus (SLE). Treatments may differ depending on the activity of the disease. If there is significant inflammation, medication aimed at reducing the inflammation will be given.

Physical therapy (PT) and maintaining a regular exercise program are important aspects of treatment for several reasons. First, if joints are painful, there is a tendency to avoid using painful parts of the body. In time, because of lack of use, these joints become dry, stiff, and less able to function. Also, muscles that are not used become weaker and lose actual muscle mass. Treatment aimed at reducing inflammation, good pain management, and active PT and exercise will help to keep affected body parts healthy and functional.

A child with arthritis will often experience pain during PT, which may make him afraid and unwilling to continue. If this happens, it is important to explain to him the difference between "good pain" and "bad pain." Good pain is that which a child feels when he pushes his body to do a little more than it did before. Any new activity, such as starting a new sport, can cause pain, especially if the child is using muscles that he had never used as vigorously. However, the pain typically lessens as the child becomes more physically active. This is different from bad pain, which continues long after the PT sessions or exercise. Chronic pain is bad pain. It does not serve any purpose and should be treated. I typically recommend Iyengar yoga for the children, adolescents, and young adults whom I treat who have arthritis. (For more on yoga, see "A Young Man with

Arthritis," below, as well as Chapter 8, "Complementary and Alternative Therapies.")

If your child has arthritis, she should not have to suffer with chronic pain. There are medications for chronic pain stemming from arthritis. (For more on medications used for the pain of arthritis, see Chapter 7, "Medicines for Treating Chronic Pain," pages 153–154.) Fortunately, more pediatric rheumatologists are becoming experts in pediatric chronic pain management. In fact, of all pediatricians, pediatric rheumatologists typically have the most expertise in understanding and treating chronic pain. Sometimes treating arthritis involves trial and error. If one medication is not working effectively, the rheumatologist may have to increase the dose or change medications. Work together with your child's doctor until the pain is under better control.

If your rheumatologist seems stuck in terms of what to do to help your child, you can suggest that he or she contact a pediatric pain specialist to get help. I often receive calls or e-mails from physicians for advice on pain management. There is also a lot of information on pain management and arthritis available to parents on the Internet from the many arthritis organizations.

A Young Man with Arthritis

Luke, a young man now in his late twenties, describes what it was like when he was diagnosed with JRA and what has helped him since.

• • •

My juvenile rheumatoid arthritis was diagnosed when I was 12 years years old. My symptoms ranged from fevers, joint pain, and stiffness to weight loss, chest pain, anemia, and joint damage. I wish I could say that I am exaggerating, but rheumatoid arthritis is simply a miserable disease with no cure whatsoever.

Rheumatoid arthritis is a chronic autoimmune disease that can affect anyone at anytime in their life. Because it is systemic, it can affect the entire body, including the organs, glands, the lymphatic system, and the joints and muscles. Unfortunately, I suffered through all of these symptoms. I took high levels of medication for years because the inflammation in my body just wouldn't go away.

When I turned 18, my symptoms suddenly went away. I was able to go to college and at least live my life on my own terms. But when I turned 23, the disease and all of its symptoms came back. That is when I realized I could either be a victim or be strong and find as many ways as possible to keep myself healthy. I tried different drugs, homeopathics, physical therapy, and even acupuncture, but nothing really worked.

I struggled for more than 10 years to find ways to live with this disease. The only answer anyone ever came up with was to just take more medication. I've learned firsthand that this is really no answer. I had just about given up when one day my doctor suggested I try practicing yoga. My first instinct was to laugh. No way could this ancient practice possibly help me. Miraculously, knock on wood, I have been in remission for almost 5 years. I don't think it is a coincidence that this is also how long I have been practicing Iyengar yoga. I know for a fact that Iyengar yoga is controlling my symptoms and controlling my disease. I have no idea what I would do without it.

Another hurdle I have to overcome is the psychological impact the disease has had on my life. I have to really listen to my body and figure out what my body needs. Ultimately, I have to learn to distinguish between good pain and bad pain and learn to trust my instincts.

I know the disease will never go away, but for the first time, I feel like I can at least control my symptoms. This is the greatest gift I have ever received. I know I'm going to be faced with more challenges in life that will seem too hard to handle. My first instinct will probably be to run and hide. But maybe, for just an instant, I can stop and remember what I've learned from yoga: that with hard work, trust, and discipline, life and all of its problems might just get better. Obviously, I wish I never had had rheumatoid arthritis. Obviously, I wish I didn't have to sit and wonder if and when it will ever come back. But I can't. Instead, I am at least going to look for ways to deal with this disease.

DISEASES ASSOCIATED WITH PAIN VERSUS CHRONIC PAIN CONDITIONS

In this chapter, I have used several diseases to illustrate how chronic pain develops and how certain factors can increase the pain. The next chapter covers chronic pain conditions. There is a subtle but important distinction between *diseases that can be associated with pain* and *chronic pain conditions*. Diseases that can be associated with pain are illnesses where the pain originally stems from a known cause such as an infection, inflammation, injury, or obstruction associated with a disease. Chronic pain conditions are illnesses where the cause of the pain (whether headaches or muscle pain) is dysfunctional pain signaling and/or muscle contractions rather than a specific structural or inflammatory cause.

{ CHAPTER THREE }

Chronic Pain Conditions

When the head aches, all members partake of the pains.
—CERVANTES

The pain started suddenly, when I was nine, as a slight pain in my knee that kept getting worse and worse. I went to an orthopedic surgeon near where I lived and had an MRI. They found a slight tear in the cartilage, and the doctor decided to operate. It was successful at first. It was a slight arthroscopic surgery, and I thought I would be back on my feet in no time. But as I went to physical therapy, the pain started getting worse. I kept pushing myself. My parents didn't know what to think. The doctor implied that I had a low pain tolerance and that I didn't want to work hard to get better.

The pain was getting worse and was affecting my sleep. I was having trouble walking. The pain was a burning sensation, like my leg was on fire. I couldn't straighten my leg because the pain was so intense. It finally stayed like that. The muscles in my ankle had atrophied and couldn't hold me up. I was starting the fifth grade, trying to do normal things, but the pain was so great that I couldn't concentrate. I was going to school only half days because of physical therapy.

I was becoming really depressed. I was losing hope. I was in so much pain, I didn't know what to do about it. I wasn't going to school normally; I didn't have any friends. It was so horrible at that age to see everyone else run around, and I couldn't. I was taking a lot of pain medication. I was also taking antianxiety pills. Nothing was really helping.

And then, I don't know how to describe it, but it's like you're traveling up a hill and you don't think you are ever going to get to the top and then you finally just reach the peak and things start happening. By the middle of sixth grade, I was out of the wheelchair and back on crutches. It took a long process to get to that point. It started by taking a step on the crutches and then I'd sit back in the wheelchair. Once I was vertical again on the crutches, that really helped.

I don't know how I originally damaged my knee. It started out as just an ache and then grew worse and worse. I was limping. There had been some torn cartilage, but I probably could have done without surgery. Today, my right leg is curved and the calf is smaller, and sometimes walking long distances is difficult. I have arthritis in my leg and hips. But I am in college now and am able to live a full and active life.

•   •   •

Childhood is not necessarily a pain-free time. There are the unavoidable aches and pains from falling off a bike and skinning a knee. Children get earaches, chicken pox, flu, and stomachaches and may even have their tonsils removed. These are all acute pain problems that go away when the infection is gone or the injury is healed. However, in this book, I am concerned with the less common but more severe pains that some children suffer from—chronic or recurrent pain that doesn't just go away.

In the previous chapter, I discussed several diseases associated with chronic pain. In this chapter, I focus on chronic pain conditions that are *functional* in nature, including chronic headaches, abdominal pain, fibromyalgia, musculoskeletal pain conditions (e.g., back or neck pain), and severe pain in one focal area of the body, known as CRPS (or RSD). *Functional* means that there is no structural, inflammatory, injury, metabolic, or other "disease"-related reasons for the pain. In other words, the pain problem relates to the function of muscles, organs, or nervous system rather than the muscles, organs, or nerves themselves being "broken" or diseased.

If symptoms such as belly pain, diarrhea, constipation, bloating, nausea, and vomiting are related to an actual inflammation in the small or large intestines, they should go away by reducing and eliminating the inflammation with steroids and other anti-inflammatory drugs. However, if the intestines are normal (without inflammation, injury, or infection) and the same symptoms are present, then something else is causing the symptoms: disordered signaling in the nervous system. When this occurs, the sensory nerves become hypersensitive and bombard the brain with pain signals. The normal pain-control mechanisms are overloaded and the child develops a functional pain disorder.

For example, in myofascial (musculoskeletal) pain, the problem is not a diseased set of muscles but rather that the muscles are extremely tense. Little tender points develop in the muscles, and tight muscles hurt! It's like having a chronic charley horse or muscle cramp in your leg. Depending on the muscles affected, symptoms include headache, backache, or pain in other areas of the body.

As a medical student, I thought *functional* meant that nothing was wrong and that the problem was "in the patient's head." I now know that I was wrong, but I wonder how many others still think that this is the definition of *functional*.

The first chronic pain condition we explore below is headaches. Chronic headache is among the most common pain problems I encounter in my clinic. I use headache to illustrate how I evaluate children who come to me with a history of chronic pain. With only a few exceptions (such as different medications or tests), the evaluation and treatment of chronic pain conditions are the same.

HEADACHES

The common misconception is that headaches are an adult disease, but some 20% of children between the ages of 5 and 17 experience chronic headaches. If the headaches are mild, even if they occur once or twice a week, they may be easily relieved with a pain reliever such as Tylenol. However, headaches that last a long time, don't get better rapidly with nonprescription (over-the-counter) medication, and begin to hamper your child's daily activities should be considered a pain problem.

It is not the number of headaches but rather how much they bother the child, especially if they start impeding sleep, eating, activities, or school, that is the true test of whether they are chronic. Some children are debilitated by one or two headaches a week, whereas others find headaches to be minor nuisances until they start coming daily or the pain continues throughout the day.

•   •   •

Danny is a 12-year-old boy who developed headaches that got worse and worse and did not respond to any pain medication. He was unable to sleep or go to school. He was hospitalized and, after MRI showed normal results, Danny underwent multiple tests, including several lumbar punctures (LPs—needles placed in his back to get cerebrospinal fluid to check for meningitis and to check the pressure of the fluid). Because the doctors had technical difficulties during the first two LPs, they performed a third. The test results all came back normal, but Danny's pain was no better.

Frustrated, the doctors began to wonder if Danny was increasing his pain complaints to get attention and decided to refer him to our pain clinic because the referring physicians knew we had psychologists as part of our program. During Danny's evaluation, we discovered symptoms of a generalized anxiety disorder and other factors that had initiated the headaches, which were then made significantly worse by the medical traumas Danny underwent in the attempt to get a diagnosis. These medical traumas actually led to PTSD, further aggravating Danny's pain problem.

• • •

This story illustrates that a detailed medical history at the start could have revealed factors that were causing Danny's headaches or at least have indicated what was making them worse. Invasive medical tests should not be the first approach, because many medical tests have risks. Doctors often forget to ask about risk factors, such as past traumas, or don't evaluate children for anxiety, learning disabilities, and other problems that affect pain.

Suppose that, for example, your daughter has been having headaches every other day and she's been missing school. You know she's in a lot of pain, but you can't figure out why she's having the headaches. There seems to be no pattern to them—sometimes they come on in the morning, sometimes at night, and there doesn't seem to be a connection to what she eats or drinks or to the amount of sleep she gets. You are stymied, and the headaches continue. What's causing them, and what can you do?

The first step is to make sure that your daughter doesn't have the type of headache that is caused by something structural in the brain (e.g., tumor, traumatic brain injury), chemical (e.g., monosodium glutamate

[MSG] reactions), or identifiable causes that can be readily treated if diagnosed (e.g., sinus infection, poor vision).

Because children's headaches have many possible causes, you should have your child evaluated by her pediatrician or family physician if the headaches seem to persist (e.g., missing two consecutive days of school because of the headache). A complete history that includes questions about other symptoms and a medical, social, and family history, as well as a thorough physical exam by a doctor, should identify the reason for most headaches.

Conditions that need to be taken care of quickly, such as a brain tumor, meningitis, or bleeding in the head (from trauma or a leaky blood vessel from a vascular malformation) should be readily apparent by how sick your child looks. If your child has unusual or sudden symptoms or signs such as fever, morning vomiting, visual disturbances, seizures; a body part with paralysis, weakness, loss of sensation, or shaking; or any sudden changes in alertness, speech, or thinking, especially after head trauma, bring him to the doctor or ER immediately.

Most other reasons for headaches do not need such urgent attention. For example, with a sinus infection, pain and tenderness can be felt when you press over the sinus areas (e.g., forehead, behind the eyes, cheeks), especially after a cold. In this case, decongestants and antibiotics will clear the headaches, and mild analgesics such as ibuprofen should help your child feel better. Sometimes allergies or changes in barometric pressure can cause headaches related to fluid or fluid shifts in the sinus cavities. Caffeine, MSG, and tannins in foods, as well as allergies to certain foods, also can trigger headaches. All of these causes should be readily identifiable. What I review in more detail here are the more common—but less easy to identify and treat—reasons for chronic headaches:

- **Headaches occurring after head injury** are often called central or postconcussion headaches and often feel as if the head is pounding or is being squeezed tightly from inside. These can last for several months after a head injury.

- **Sensory overload headaches** can be caused by strong odors, loud noises, bright lights, sun poisoning, or drinking a cold liquid too quickly—in other words, "too much" of any sensory experience can cause headaches in children. Some children are more sensitive to intense sensory exposure than others. (See Chapter 6, "Pervasive Developmental Disorders," for more on sensory exposure in children with autism spectrum disorders and Asperger's syndrome.)

- **Myofascial or tension headaches** (often called **chronic daily headaches** by neurologists) are caused by muscle tenseness (contraction) in the scalp, neck, shoulders, or face. They typically feel like pressure or heavy or squeezing pain at the back of the head or all over the head. They often develop on top of other headaches, such as migraines. When migraines start lasting throughout the day or feel like they are coming very frequently, and especially if the usual medicines used for migraines are not working, then the main reason for your child's headaches is likely myofascial (muscles in spasm). Almost any treatment that stretches the muscles and relaxes the CNS will work for these headaches.

- **Temporomandibular Joint (TMJ) headaches** (often called **facial pain headaches**) are most often caused by a malalignment of the teeth and jaw. The TMJ is the joint located right in front of the ears where the jaw attaches to the head. Teeth clenching or bite abnormalities that put abnormal pressure on the TMJ during chewing can produce both facial pain and TMJ headaches, which are often felt as throbbing, aching, or pressure at the temples but can lead to myofascial headaches throughout the head.

- **Vision-related headaches** are caused by strain on eye muscles related to poor vision (e.g., squinting to see the blackboard) or binocular fusion problems, where each eye sees the same object in slightly different locations (meaning the vision from each eye doesn't fuse into a single clear picture). These headaches may be located around and behind the eyes and can lead to myofascial headaches.

- **Migraine headaches** are often what I hear parents call almost all types of problematic headaches in children. Most turn out to be myofascial/tension headaches. Migraines usually occur on one side of the head in adults, but not necessarily so in children. There is usually an aura, meaning that the person sees spots, flashes, or other signals before the onset of a migraine. The migraine itself is usually accompanied by sensitivity to light and sound and may also be associated with nausea and vomiting. Most children just want to try to sleep during a bad migraine. The best way to treat migraines is to prevent them with stress-management techniques (see Chapter 10, "Helping Your Child Cope with Chronic Pain"), exercise, a healthy diet that avoids foods that trigger migraines for your child, and preventive medications if needed. Simple migraines can be diagnosed and treated by most child neurologists. If they are hard to treat, consider tension headaches and other factors that may be keeping the migraines going (see Chapter 5, "Factors That Contribute to Chronic Pain").

Deciding whether to take your child to the doctor for treatment of headaches depends on the type of headaches, how much they are bothering your child, and how much they are getting in the way of your child's normal life, especially if your child is missing school or finding it hard to do schoolwork because of them.

Some children start getting headaches even before they master language. Toddlers with a headache may cry, turn pale, vomit, or bang their heads. This wide range of symptoms and behaviors can make it difficult for a parent to know what is wrong.

The initial history that your child's primary care physician takes, which should include a combination of medical, psychological, social, and family questions, will help her to decide if the headaches are the result of a known cause that can be readily treated (e.g., sinus infection, tension headaches, vision problems) or if more tests are needed (e.g., sinus x-rays, computed tomography [CT] scan or brain MRI, blood count).

However, if the test results are negative yet the headaches do not get better with treatment and your child is unable to return to his normal activities, a further assessment is needed to determine what is causing the chronic headaches and to identify a treatment plan. Below are some typical questions that I would ask if I were evaluating your child. It is useful to think about the answers to these questions before seeking medical help to identify the possible source(s) of the headaches. This will help your child's primary care physician to come up with a treatment plan more quickly.

I might ask the following questions to learn about the nature of the headaches and how they are getting in the way of daily life:

- How long has your child been bothered by the headaches?
- Did a head injury, infection, dental work, or other event, such as attending a new school, precede the headaches?
- Does the headache occur at any particular time of day (e.g., when the child first awakens), week (e.g., school days only), or month (with menses, for girls)?
- How often does it occur, and how long does it last?
- Does it come on suddenly or gradually?
- Is it preceded by any aura (visual changes, spots, sounds, or other unusual feelings)?
- Where is the pain located, and what does it feel like (e.g., pounding, stabbing)?
- What makes it worse, and what helps it feel better?

- What medications (name, dose, how often, and for how long) has your child taken for her headaches, and what is she still taking (and do they help)?
- What herbs or nondrug therapies has your child tried for the headaches (e.g., warm baths, ice packs, listening to music, PT, massage, yoga, relaxation training, hypnotherapy, acupuncture, psychotherapy)? Did they help?
- What does the pain stop your child from doing (e.g., concentrating, doing homework, attending school, playing sports, attending social activities with friends, participating in activities with family)?
- Does the pain interfere with falling asleep or staying asleep? Does your child wake up feeling tired/not rested?
- Does the pain affect your child's appetite? Has she lost or gained weight because of the headaches?
- What do you think is causing the headaches?

COMPLEX REGIONAL PAIN SYNDROME TYPE I

CRPS type I (or CRPS-I, formerly known as RSD) is a debilitating painful disorder of a part of the body, often one or both of the extremities (although it can be anywhere on the body). Pain may occur after a minor injury or surgery but also may occur without an obvious prior event. The pain is often described as a burning, squeezing, or stabbing/shooting pain.

The hallmarks of CRPS are supersensitivity to even light touch in the affected area, the type of pain noted above, and interference with the use of the leg or arm if that is the part affected. Sometimes, there are swelling and color changes (red/blue). There may be skin and hair changes from lack of touch to that body part. The muscles may weaken and shrink from nonuse. Below, two children describe what CRPS feels like to them:

•   •   •

I sometimes feel like someone is taking a torch of fire to my ankle when I walk on it; it feels like a lightning bolt is going up my leg. Sometimes when I bend or move, it feels like it is going to explode. It is so sensitive that I can't wear my jeans and I have to wear baggy pants all of the time. If someone tries to touch my leg during physical therapy, I go through the roof in sharp, excruciating pain. Or even if someone accidentally bangs my knee, it seems to be worse for the rest of the day.

*　　*　　*

If I had to describe the pain in my leg, I might describe it as numb, but I really don't think that's quite right. It's not numb like you get with epidurals. First, there is the lack of its feeling stable, because of a pins-and-needles feeling, which is really disturbing, and it doesn't want to move normally, and won't take my weight, and then there is a circulation-being-cut-off kind of numbness. I get shooting pains, but not all the time. Most of the time, my leg seriously aches, feels like it's being crushed, and generally being eaten up from the inside. (I know that sounds strange, but it's a description I developed a while ago for this cold burning kind of feeling.)

*　　*　　*

The painful body part is often sensitive to light touch; even a brush of clothing, water, or a light breeze can be excruciatingly painful, and any contact with that sensitive area (such as someone accidentally bumping it) can cause more severe pain. A child with CRPS-I may not want to wear shoes or have the sheets touch that part of her body at night, which may lead to sleep problems. Because the child is often afraid of someone touching the painful body part, she may attempt to avoid school or other social events. Additionally, the painful body part might become sensitive to temperature (either heat or cold). As the pain worsens, patients have difficulty moving the limb, which can lead to stiffness and more pain. These symptoms can also come and go.

The prevalence of CRPS-I tends to be higher in adolescents, although it can appear in younger children. As with many other chronic pain conditions (e.g., migraines, IBS, fibromyalgia, and facial pain), CRPS-I seems to be more prevalent in girls than in boys. Dancers, athletes, and gymnasts are at greater risk of CRPS-I. And, as with other chronic pain conditions, many children with CRPS-I tend to be bright, high-achieving, and perfectionistic and have other factors, such as a previously unsuspected learning disability or an anxiety disorder, that can keep the pain going.

CRPS-I is caused by an abnormal turn-on in the sensory nervous system, not only in the affected body part but also all along the sensory nerve pathway up the spine and into the brain. The most common approach to treating CRPS-I in children and adolescents is educating them about the condition and what can be done to make it better or worse. Physical therapy is aimed at getting the child used to touching, using, and strengthening the affected body part. In fact, moving and using the affected body part is the key to turning down the volume on the pain and turning off the brain pain messages. I always remind a child that even if he feels more pain initially with PT, it does not mean he is causing more injury.

A Child with Complex Regional Pain Syndrome Type I

Howard is 10-year-old with JRA. His rheumatologist referred him to me because Howard was having significant pain in his legs and other joints despite treatment for seven months with strong anti-inflammatory drugs (steroids, methotrexate, and nonsteroidal anti-inflammatory drugs [NSAIDs]). He hurt so much that he was unable to engage in PT. He refused to go to school because he said he was in too much pain, had difficulty standing, and couldn't walk or even sit at his desk through a day at school.

Howard was falling behind in school. He was becoming less active, and his legs were getting weaker and his joints stiffer. The lack of PT added to further joint deterioration. Also, Howard was depressed.

When I first met Howard, he was in a wheelchair. After getting a history of his problems and his pain, I examined him and found that the skin on his legs, from his knees to his toes, was extremely sensitive to even light touch. He feared getting bumped or even touched. He said that it was difficult for him to sleep at night because contact with the covers and sheets worsened the pain.

•   •   •

This type of pain (burning, extreme sensitivity to light touch of the skin) was not the type of pain that children with arthritis have. Arthritis pain would have responded to the increased anti-inflammatory medication prescribed by Howard's rheumatologist. Rather, Howard had neuropathic (nerve) pain that probably had little to do with his arthritis. I diagnosed his condition as CRPS-I. Howard did not remember injuring himself when the pain started, but he noticed that his legs gradually became more and more sensitive to touch and that the PT he was doing for his arthritis became more painful until he couldn't do it anymore.

In addition to his depression, Howard seemed to have many characteristics of someone with an anxiety disorder. He was an only child of a single mom who worked. His absences from school and chronic pain were causing her to miss work. The health insurance for Howard's treatment was provided through her employer, and so she couldn't afford to lose her job. Howard's mom was feeling a lot of pressure and wanted Howard to get better fast—she wanted a magic pill to cure him so he could go back to school, attend PT sessions, and most of all stop complaining. She was frustrated when after only one week of treatment Howard was still in pain. She admitted to me that she felt helpless when her son cried in pain and angry with him for causing her to miss work. She also felt guilty about the anger. "What kind of person gets angry at a child who is in terrible pain?" she asked me.

First, anxiety disorders can have a genetic component. Thus, if

Mom is anxious, it is not unlikely that her son will be also. Second, kids who are sensitive, and especially an only child of a single parent, are going to monitor their parent. If they notice their parent becoming anxious, whether about work or money or the pain problem, they may become anxious, too. There is research showing that maternal anxiety is a risk factor for child anxiety and chronic pain.

Howard was very sensitive to his mother's mood and her reactions to stressors in her life. So the loop is: Single mom has lots of real-life stressors such as needing to support herself and her child and needing to keep her job so that she has insurance to pay for treatment for her son's pain problem. Son is anxious about his pain and his ability to make it through a day at school. He has trouble coping and feels out of control. He's missing school and falling behind. He starts noticing that his mother is frustrated, angry, and anxious, and this makes him more anxious. Mother's and son's anxieties begin to feed into each other. This scenario is common in families with a child with chronic pain.

I also learned, by talking to Howard's mother, that her guilt about her anger was causing her not to set normal disciplinary limits for her son. She was letting him get away with behavior, she said, that she never would have allowed had he not been in pain.

I suggested that Howard see a child psychiatry fellow in our clinic who helped him understand his fears about going to school, helped him develop a plan for getting caught up in school, and taught him some breathing and relaxation techniques and strategies to help him handle the pain and to cope when he felt anxious.

After several sessions, the child psychiatrist recommended that Howard take an SSRI (Zoloft) for his anxiety and depression to help him relax while he was learning to practice his new coping skills, which we hoped would ultimately replace the drugs to calm his anxiety and reduce his depression. I also met with his mom to help her learn how to parent a child with JRA and chronic pain. For example, I suggested that it was important for Howard to have daily routines and that she should let him know that there were things he was expected to do, such as pick up after himself at home. Control is a big issue for kids with chronic pain because they tend to feel so out of control much of the time. Therefore, many of the plans we came up with for Howard were about giving him control over some aspect of his life.

Howard's mom met with the school staff members, and together they worked out a plan for Howard to attend school in small increments that gradually increased until he was able to master a full day in school. They also developed a schedule for him to complete assignments at home for the classes he was missing.

Howard and his mom also came up with a plan of their own. Massage seemed to help Howard's pain, so for 15 minutes every night, his mom would give him a head-and-shoulder massage. It started out as a reward for Howard's increasing his amount of physical activity that day, but it became a nightly routine that both Howard and his mom enjoyed. The massages relaxed his muscles and tension, gave Howard and his mom a special routine together before bed, and also helped him fall asleep.

They also set up a plan of rewards for Howard's accomplishments. For example, when he was able to stay in school for two periods a day for a week, they would go to a favorite burger restaurant. They set up a series of positive reinforcements of this type, each predicated on Howard's mastering a new task. When Howard was finally able to stay in school all day for an entire week, his reward was a trip to the mall (without his wheelchair) to pick out a new video.

To help Howard cope with his fear of pain during PT, I prescribed a short-acting opioid (oxycodone) as a brief but strong pain-control medication so that he could gradually increase the work that he did in PT. The physical therapist and Howard worked out a plan for increasing the amount of exercises he could do. As he became more confident in his abilities, he no longer needed the medication. I also recommended that

Howard learn Iyengar yoga. Today Howard credits yoga with producing the most dramatic physical results, because it made him feel strong and competent.

Within three to four months of following the program we had set up, Howard was able to practice his yoga poses at home, attend yoga class and PT once a week, and attend school full-time. He had begun playing outdoors with neighborhood friends and was more physically active. His anxiety disorder was under control; he no longer felt worried and anxious all the time. His depression had also lifted and his mood was more upbeat.

CHILDHOOD FIBROMYALGIA

When Timmy became ill and didn't get well, at first, as his mother, I just wanted to know that whatever it was wasn't life-threatening. Of course, cancer was my biggest fear. No one could come up with a definitive diagnosis. Timmy had a low-grade fever all the time and was listless, lethargic, cold, and pale; had poor appetite; and went from sore throats to headaches and then to abdominal pains. Each school year, he would get a virus and not get well entirely. The acute illness would abate and then he would have a low-grade fever with either a minor sore throat or headache for another week or so, and he always looked sick around the eyes, and always pale and cold. Then, when he returned to school, he would be fine for weeks or a month and then get what seemed to be a virus and would go through the same thing; out of school for three or four days at a time.

He never struck me as lazy, depressed, or school-phobic. When he was feeling well, he would be very active—involved in sports and very social. When he didn't feel well, he didn't want to do anything. I wasn't thinking of a pain syndrome; it never occurred to me. Once I was presented with the diagnosis, I had mixed reactions. I was greatly relieved that it wasn't cancer or any other horrendous diagnosis. But having been diagnosed with chronic fatigue syndrome and then fibromyalgia eight years ago myself, I was not thrilled. I thought: *Chronic fatigue syndrome and fibromyalgia—oh no, not at ten years.*

• • •

Until recently, fibromyalgia, a disease characterized by chronic widespread pain in the fibrous tissues of the muscles, ligaments, and tendons and fatigue ranging from mild to severe and symptoms that could change by the hour, has been poorly understood and commonly misdiagnosed. Fibromyalgia sufferers were left to doubt themselves as doctors struggled to pin down the condition. In children, fibromyalgia is often mistakenly diagnosed as growing pains or behavioral problems, and it is commonly mistaken for chronic fatigue syndrome because the symptoms of the two conditions are similar and may even be variations of the same condition.

Although there is increasing research on adult fibromyalgia, less is known about juvenile fibromyalgia (hereafter referred to simply as fibromyalgia), as it is called in children and adolescents, despite the fact that it is a common pediatric chronic pain syndrome. After a series of blood tests performed to look for other rheumatologic disorders produce negative or mildly positive results, many doctors are baffled. However, the diagnosis can be made positively if the child has a history of widespread pain and numerous tender points throughout the body.

I do not find it necessary to label a child as having fibromyalgia unless I think that giving a specific diagnosis will be helpful for insurance purposes or similar reasons. Many parents, especially those who have fibromyalgia themselves, will interpret from their own experience or reading that fibromyalgia is a lifelong illness and there is no cure. This is incorrect. Juvenile fibromyalgia is quite curable. I also think that believing they have an "incurable illness" does more to harm children than does the condition itself.

Fibromyalgia is characterized by an extremely aroused CNS, and this is why it can be associated with chronic fatigue, sleep disturbances, pain all over the body, and other neural imbalance problems such as IBS and tension headaches. Sometimes, as with chronic fatigue syndrome, the fibromyalgia symptoms begin with a viral illness, but the flulike symptoms remain after the infection has cleared.

Although we still know relatively little about what causes fibromyalgia, we are learning more about its symptoms. For example, we know that the flulike symptoms that are common in patients with fibromyalgia are caused by proteins called proinflammatory cytokines. These proteins are produced by immune cells (lymphocytes) that respond to viral infections. When the levels of these cytokines are increased, they can cause fatigue and sleep disturbances. If the body is deprived of restorative, deep sleep, it starts to break down so that bodily systems don't work as well: Thinking can be impaired (sometimes called fibrofog), physical and emotional exhaustion can develop, and depression ensues.

We also know that the immune cells "talk" with nerves that carry pain signals, and each influences the other. The activation of the immune cells and the pain signals can cause depression, anxiety, fatigue, sleep problems, weakness, and widespread pain. Because the CNS is so out of balance, this imbalance can spread to the brain–gut nervous system and cause IBS symptoms as well as to muscles, causing myofascial headaches and other pains, all of which are symptoms associated with fibromyalgia.

As with other pain conditions described in this chapter, the primary treatments include increasing function with exercise, restoring CNS balance (for example, with yoga or acupuncture), reducing stress, and increasing relaxation.

FUNCTIONAL BOWEL DISORDERS

In the previous chapter, I described IBDs that can be associated with abdominal pain and that have an identifiable cause—the inflammation. In this chapter, I discuss functional bowel disorders, the cluster of conditions associated with abdominal pain in which there is a *functional* cause. Functional bowel disorders are identified by belly pain with or without other gastrointestinal (GI) symptoms and are *not* associated with inflammatory, metabolic, or structural abnormality of the intestinal tract. The pain or symptoms are caused by abnormal nerve signaling between the brain and the intestines, which makes the intestines hypersensitive and may result in increased pain.

The most common of the functional bowel disorders associated with belly pain are:

- **Functional abdominal pain (FAP)**, in which there is diffuse, all-around-the-belly pain without any other gastrointestinal symptoms.
- **Functional dyspepsia**, in which there is pain in the esophagus and/or stomach area and the pain feels like an ulcer (burning in one spot in the middle at the base of the chest) or like acid reflux (burning in the chest itself).
- **IBS**, in which there is widespread belly pain that might move around the belly, as in FAP, but there are also other gastrointestinal symptoms, such as nausea, vomiting, bloating, constipation, and/or diarrhea. Some children with IBS have belly pain with cramping and diarrhea. These children may avoid going to school, fearing they may have an episode of diarrhea that would embarrass them in front of their friends. This fear actually increases the sensitivity of the intestines and can make both the belly pain and the diarrhea worse. Some children with IBS have constipation. Others may have both diarrhea and constipation at various times.

As described in Chapter 1 ("What Is Pain?"), the sympathetic (fight or flight) branch of the ANS and the stress hormone system can affect pain sensitivity. In functional bowel disorders, children's intestines become very sensitive to anything inside them. However, because there is nothing wrong with the intestines themselves, the results for common tests that are performed or ordered by the gastroenterologist come back negative.

The problem is in the nerves that carry signals between the brain and the intestines (what I call the brain–gut axis). The volume of these signals is increased (turned up) in these belly pain conditions. Even very small signals are magnified. Normally we cannot feel our stomach grumble with hunger, the physical sensation of swallowing small amounts of food, or intestinal gas. However, when a child has a functional bowel disorder, this normal intestinal activity can become incredibly painful. When this happens, the child may develop conditioned food aversions: Because the gut is so sensitive, certain foods that she normally ate without a reaction now become associated with pain (even if the actual foods themselves are not responsible for the pain). Children begin to avoid those foods or even stop eating to reduce the frequency of the belly pain attacks (because they think the cause of the pain is the food rather than their brain–gut nerve signals). This food avoidance typically doesn't work.

It is not that their stomachs can't tolerate that food or that they have a food allergy. Rather it is because their brain learns quickly to make a new association (new connections) between that food and belly pain. Once their brains have made this food–pain connection, some children will actually develop belly pain when they eat those foods. This is called a learned or conditioned response. Russian scientist Pavlov taught his dog that every time a bell rang, he would get something to eat. After a while, the dog would salivate just at the sound of the bell, even when he didn't receive food. It is the same with these children; they learn to develop belly pain because they believe that the food will cause them pain. When the child's nervous system is calmed down and balanced again so that it is not so sensitive, the child is able to eat those foods that she previously avoided without any stomach pain. It is not uncommon for a viral flu to set off this disordered nerve signaling and the functional bowel disorder, and cause pain and other GI symptoms.

Functional bowel disorders can be diagnosed without a lot of tests and medical procedures. The child's medical and family history and the physical exam are typically the keys to a diagnosis, with only a few exceptions. (For example, to diagnose functional dyspepsia, both acid reflux and stomach ulcers must be ruled out.)

I don't believe that there is any set time period or severity that must be present before a diagnosis of a functional bowel disorder can be made. If the pain bothers the child and/or gets in the way of normal daily activities, sleep, or healthy eating, then the problem needs to be treated. The goal of treatment is to get the brain–gut nervous system regulated. Just as with fibromyalgia and other chronic pain conditions, treatment includes promoting restorative sleep, exercise, and healthy eating and encouraging the child to return to a normal life.

I am often surprised by how many pediatric gastroenterologists know how to diagnose a functional bowel disorder such as IBS yet do not offer effective treatment, other than reassurance that "nothing is wrong" or that the condition is "stress related." (In Appendix B, "Pediatric Pain and Gastrointestinal Pain Programs," on page 273, I have listed pediatric gastroenterology programs that have indicated that they use a mind–body approach to treating children with these pain disorders and have extensive experience in both diagnosing and treating children with functional bowel disorders.)

Certain medications are used in functional bowel disorders for constipation-predominant IBS (such as Zelnorm) and diarrhea-predominant IBS (such as Elavil in low doses, starting with 10 mg at night). Constipation also can be treated with herbal remedies (apricot and linnem), sorbitol (candies for diabetic people), MiraLax, and stool softeners such as Colace. Diarrhea can also be helped by Immodium as a temporary measure. For children with symptoms of anxiety and IBS, studies have shown that Celexa, an SSRI, can be effective. Finally, peppermint-oil geltabs before meals can be effective in reducing belly pain, and ginger taken in the form of ginger candy or dried sweetened ginger or tea brewed with pieces of fresh ginger can reduce nausea.

However, typically medications alone do not work with functional bowel disorders associated with reduced function. A treatment plan that combines drugs and nondrug therapies is usually the most successful. Examples of nondrug therapies include Iyengar yoga, hypnotherapy, acupuncture, and others. (For a detailed discussion of these therapies, see Chapter 8, "Complementary and Alternative Therapies.") These and other similar treatments help to calm the CNS, rebalance chemicals in the brain, and teach the child self-help tools to calm his own nervous system and alter pain signaling. Below is the story of a patient of mine with typical IBS.

A Child with Irritable Bowel Syndrome

JoAnn is a 13-year-old who, about six months before coming to see me, had developed belly pain associated with some intermittent constipation, diarrhea, bloating, and nausea. She had had GERD early on, but this had stopped. These symptoms continued and worsened until she was having significant abdominal cramping and diarrhea every morning. Soon she was regularly missing the entire morning at school. She began to restrict what she ate and developed rigid food preferences because she feared that certain foods would cause her diarrhea.

JoAnn also began having trouble falling asleep at night, although once she was asleep, she remained asleep. She started limiting her social activities because of the diarrhea and because she was not feeling well. She said that nothing helped and eating made her belly pain worse. JoAnn originally saw a pediatric gastroenterologist, who performed an endoscopy (a procedure where a tube is used to examine and take biopsies of the esophagus, stomach, and small intestine), which produced normal findings. He recommended that JoAnn see a psychiatrist, explaining that this was a "stress-related condition."

A few months after the belly pains began, JoAnn had seen a psychologist for three visits for grief counseling after her grandmother's sudden death. Four months later, she was evaluated by a second pediatric gastroenterologist and she was given Elavil. She was referred by that gastroenterologist to our Pediatric Pain Program after the Elavil failed to relieve her pain.

JoAnn described her belly pain as "throbbing, stabbing, cramping," and often associated with sore abdominal muscles. She rated the pain on a scale of 0 to 10 (in which 10 is the worst pain possible) as averaging a 6, with a range from 2 to 8. She reported intermittent diarrhea and constipation and said that the problems related to reflux and bloating were gone, but she still had occasional nausea. She was no longer vomiting. She had previously been given a number of medications, including Tigan for nausea, Elavil, Bentyl, Immodium, stool softeners, fiber, and Mylanta.

• • •

Reviewing JoAnn's symptoms with her, I learned that she had general fatigue. She had headaches at least once a week that were helped by Tylenol. She had occasional trouble breathing, heart palpitations, and tightness in the throat from panic attacks. She had some dizziness when standing and occasional hot and cold flashes. The belly pain attacks occurred about once a week. JoAnn's mom reported no significant medical history other than as described above.

JoAnn still got A's and B's, even though she had been missing every morning of school for about six months. JoAnn's physical examination findings were normal except for some slight belly tenderness near the bottom at the right. She reported having trouble concentrating, feeling lonely, and crying often. She said that she had been having panic attacks for the last three to four months, although she was "used to them" and recognized that they were "stress-related." She said that she was most stressed out by homework and by pressure to be at school when she was sick. She admitted that she was a "worrier."

As a result of what I learned about JoAnn and in the physical exam, I diagnosed her conditions as (1) IBS with constipation and diarrhea, abdominal pain, and nausea; (2) myofascial (muscle-spasm) headaches; (3) major depressive disorder, in partial remission; and (4) recent-onset panic attacks.

One thing that made JoAnn anxious was that she might have an attack during school and might not be able to get to the bathroom. This is a common concern for children with IBS. "Access to bathrooms may be an obstacle to attending school," says Lynn Walker, Ph.D., director of the Division of Adolescent Medicine and Behavior Science at Vanderbilt University Medical Center. "For many of these children, going to the bathroom provides symptom relief. However, they may be reluctant to use the bathroom because of privacy concerns, inadequate time between classes, or teasing by classmates." Dr. Walker suggests that "parents can ask their physician to write a letter to the school requesting that their child be allowed to use the bathroom as needed, without asking to be excused or waiting for a break between classes. Often just knowing that this is possible reduces children's anxiety so much that their symptoms are reduced. I have never had a child take advantage of this arrangement to get out of class."

I recommended two medications to treat JoAnn's IBS. The first was Mellaril, a drug that would quiet down her nervous system rapidly and help ease the panic and belly pain. This was planned as a short-term solution while the next medication had time to take effect. The other medication was Celexa, an SSRI that has been shown to be effective in children with IBS. I told JoAnn that she could use Immodium for diarrhea and

MiraLax for constipation. We talked at length about cognitive therapies such as hypnosis or biofeedback and PTs such as yoga or massage. Also, I encouraged her to get more exercise and recommended swimming and walking. We discussed her diet and reviewed what a healthy diet was, and I recommended that she try to eat fewer greasy and fatty foods.

Finally, I referred her to a psychologist who was skilled in cognitive-behavioral therapy so that JoAnn could learn some skills to reduce her CNS sensitivity, calm her body and her mind, and reduce her feelings of panic and her pain. I asked her to come back in a month to see how this plan was working. When I saw JoAnn again, she was doing much better and, after six months of treatment, she was taking only the SSRI, no longer had belly pain or panic attacks, was attending school full-time, was active again with her friends, and was finding it much easier to concentrate on her schoolwork.

JoAnn's story is similar to the stories of many of the children and adolescents I see with chronic headaches, fibromyalgia, and other chronic pain problems. The evaluation and goals for treatment are similar in all: calm the nervous system, help your child learn to cope and function normally, and help your child's body heal. In the next chapter, I explain how children show and tell you that they are in pain.

PART II

How Much Pain Is Your Child In?

{ CHAPTER FOUR }

How Children Express Pain
and What They Mean

When I hear a baby's cry of pain change to a normal cry of hunger, to my ears, that is the most beautiful music.
—ALBERT SCHWEITZER

Louisa is three years old and has a painful form of JA. While most children begin to walk around the age of one, Louisa seemed to refuse to learn to walk. She became increasingly irritable and withdrawn. Doctors initially thought she was developmentally delayed with a difficult temperament. In reality, she was just too young to articulate the excruciating pain she felt when she tried to walk.

• • •

We all experience and express pain in different ways. Most children with chronic pain have no trouble letting us know that they are in pain. Even very young children—infants—express themselves when they are in pain. They may cry or become irritable. The child is not unsure of his pain. Rather, we as parents sometimes have difficulty trying to interpret our child's behavior and understand what he is trying to tell us.

In my pediatric training, I learned to listen to moms and dads, because they know their child best. As a parent, I learned to read subtle cues that my daughters shared with me when they were in pain. Interestingly, they were quite different from one another in their expression of pain. One daughter was very vocal and demonstrative. With her, it was difficult to know how much pain she was in because even lesser pain was displayed with all the gusto of an Academy Award–winning performance! My second daughter was a challenge, too, but in a different way; I had to pay closer attention to her physical cues because she just became quiet, withdrawn, and irritable, rarely complaining about her pain. My third daughter's pain was expressed dramatically or subtly, depending on her mood. Over time we parents learn to read our children, but there are times when we are uncertain. This chapter is intended to help you read your child.

"The teenager who is being constantly alarmed [by pain] is going to be antsy, jumpy, nervous; find it difficult to concentrate; find it difficult to remember; and find it difficult to communicate. He will become sleep deprived, take on a pain face (sunken and darkened eyes, distracted look, etc.), and generally will become what psychologists call overly vigilant," says Dr. Christopher Eccleston, director of the Pain Management Unit at the Royal National Hospital for Rheumatic Diseases in Bath, United Kingdom.

I think that as parents, we all want to do something if we see our child suffering; not doing something seems like bad parenting, not to mention cruel. But what if we do something that should make the pain better, yet there is still no change in our child's behavior? Suppose she is still crying or acting out? What if she is just quiet and withdrawn? What do these signs mean? Does it mean that the something that we did to reduce the pain worked? What was that something? As you will see throughout this book, chronic pain often responds better to less—or at least more subtle—forms of intervention.

Your understanding of your child's pain will also play a role in what type of medical treatment he gets and whether the treatment works. Doctors will differ in how well they understand and respond to your child's symptoms. Unfortunately, there is no objective test to assess pain. Pain is simply what the child feels. However, there are four general indicators of how much pain a child is in. You will learn how to recognize the signs of pain by paying attention to four things:

- What your child says
- How your child behaves or acts
- What you learn as you communicate with your child
- How your child's body reacts

WHAT SHE SAYS

Children describe their pain in many ways. Depending on a child's age, she may use words such as *achy*, *sharp*, *dull*, *electrical*, *burning*, *throbbing*, *pressure*, or *stabbing*. Such words can help you and your child's doctor understand the source of the pain and find the right treatment.

For example, this teenage girl with RSD (CRPS) describes her pain and offers lots of clues for parents and doctor:

• • •

My foot always feels painful. Whether I'm sitting, standing, or doing anything, there is constantly pain streaming up and down my leg. It feels as if thousands of tiny needles are being violently stabbed and pressed through my ankle every single second.

There are also spasms which feel like the muscles are contracting and being pulled at the same time. This usually makes me jump and is extremely painful as they come very often. It is as if my nerves are being electrocuted and my body can't do anything to stop it.

I cannot move my toes and there is little range of motion in my entire ankle and my knee. Anything touching my ankle or knee, even the slightest of pressure at any time, causes more pain to shoot through my body. A shoe, sock, or people touching my leg are all painful, but even something as light as a sheet is difficult to tolerate. It feels like the threads of the sheet have been replaced with blades of glass, scratching and digging into my skin.

Perhaps the scariest symptom of my RSD is the color changes that take place in my ankle. When the weather changes, my ankle does, too. Blue, purple, red, and other colors appear all the way up my legs from my toes to my calf when it is cold. My ankle has been almost every color I can imagine. When this is happening, the pain is stinging and burning a bit like when you have blood drawn, only much worse. Sometimes the stinging and throbbing pain builds up to the point that you feel you will scream till it eventually goes numb. This is really scary—it looks like my foot is dead or has been frozen. It won't move at all. Then suddenly, it defrosts and the pain builds up again.

When I stand up, it takes a while for me to actually be able to put any pressure whatsoever on my leg. When I do, my knee just gives out, causing me to suddenly fall over.

RSD is extremely debilitating. My toenails fall off, my hair falls out. I cannot walk or stand properly. I don't sleep, but I have no proof that I have any disease.

When I get burning pains, it is like my foot is being experimented on and I am being tortured and poked with hot sticks.

* * *

Of course, not all children, even older ones, can articulate their pain as well as this young girl. Younger children, those with cognitive or learning disabilities, or frustrated or highly distressed children, may tell you that the pain "just hurts" or they may simply groan or cry. Some children become withdrawn and quiet. In such cases, you and your child's doctor will have to learn about the pain by honing your observation and communication skills.

I remember during my residency, early in my pediatric training, a mother brought her eight-year-old daughter to see me. The mom said that her child had awakened that morning holding her belly and crying. The child had no fever, but the mom was worried that something was terribly wrong and that her child was in great pain. When I saw the child, she was curled up on her mom's lap with her head buried into her mom's side. When I asked the girl what was wrong, she just buried her head deeper. I tried to make contact by commenting that she looked pretty upset.

As a relatively new physician, I was anxious about my performance. What if the child's reticence prevented me from taking an oral history, performing a physical examination, and determining what was bothering her, where, and to what degree? It all added up to failure.

Meanwhile, the girl continued to whimper until finally, out of frustration, she yelled at me, "It just hurts!" She must have thought I was really dumb. But her outburst registered with me. How could I not know that she was suffering? She knew!

Most physicians will not have the time or intimate knowledge of your child's specific history to make the leap from "this child is complaining about something" to "I know what is causing the pain." (Because of the lack of feedback from the patient, some pediatricians joke that it feels like they are practicing veterinary medicine.) This is where your role as an advocate for your child comes in. You need to find ways to make your child's doctor understand your child's pain. If you have a good doctor, she may call on you to help your child express herself when she is in pain, interpret her pain-related behavior, and determine when pain needs medical attention or if it can be taken care of at home. If you have a less patient doctor, you may want to find another one or at least be ready to offer this information without being asked and see if you caught the doctor on a stressful day.

HOW HE ACTS

Most parents know that their child often acts different from his "normal self" when he is in pain, and there are, of course, the obvious signs that your child is in pain: crying, grimacing, groaning, or holding or rubbing his leg or stomach. But there are more subtle signs. Your child may become less active, agitated, or sleep or eat less than usual. He may show less interest in play or other activities or may just be grumpy. Thus, what the infant or child is not doing can be as important as what he is doing. How well you understand your child's pain will play a critical role in what type of medical treatment he gets and whether or not the treatment works.

Some children may magnify their behavior because they are aware that it makes their pain and suffering more believable. Thirteen-year-old Lisa told me that she avoided going to school because she was afraid that someone would accidentally bump into her. She had chronic pain in her arm that, according to Lisa, was "totally unbearable" when it was touched. When she did go to school, she avoided contact with people and cradled her arm. However, because her arm was not in a cast, bandaged, or swollen, she feared that no one would believe that she was in terrible pain because she had no "proof."

A child's response to pain may be influenced by its severity, type, location, and duration. For example, if the pain comes on quickly, is of short duration, and of high intensity, the child's reaction is likely to be more dramatic. In this case it may be easy to recognize that your child is in pain. This kind of pain is usually the result of acute injuries such as when a child breaks his arm falling off a swing at the playground. The child's behavior then may match the severity of the injury. However, with pain that is less intense but lasts longer, the child may be in pain for some time before you notice changes in his behavior. In this case, common sources of pain include headaches, achy joints, and muscle pain.

As pain becomes chronic, children often adapt by learning how to cope or deal with the pain unless their coping abilities are hindered by stress or the pain begins to escalate beyond what they can tolerate. Remember, just because a child with chronic pain is not acting the same as a child in acute pain does not mean that he is not in pain.

I am often frustrated by nurses or doctors who discount a hospitalized child's reports of pain after they see him playing Nintendo or interacting with visitors, declaring that "he doesn't seem to be in pain." Children who have chronic pain do not typically act like children with acute pain. This is because they may have adopted effective approaches to cope with their pain—under certain circumstances and for limited periods of time. The challenge for parents is to figure out what a certain behavior means, because a behavior, such as crying, can express a variety of states of mind—anger, sadness, fear, or frustration—not just pain.

Observing Your Child

Even if your child is not complaining, he may be in pain. Consider the following questions. Is your child . . .

- Limiting his/her physical activities?
- More tired than normal or having trouble sleeping?
- More argumentative or irritable than usual?
- Quieter than usual?
- Having trouble concentrating and with schoolwork?
- Eating differently?
- Not wanting to go to school?
- Having trouble with other children at school?
- Showing a change in appearance?

Although any of the above behaviors may be a sign that your child is in pain, be careful not to overattribute specific behavior changes to the pain itself—there may be other reasons why your child is acting differently. For example, a child who is sad, angry, upset, bored, hungry, or anxious might become clingy and irritable or avoid school and other social interaction.

You know your child better than anyone else. It's unreasonable to expect anyone, even your child's doctor, to know more about the causes of your child's pain than you do. Sure, the doctor may know the medical terminology and be able to prescribe the drugs and other treatments to make your child better, but you are the one who sees how your child acts on a daily basis.

WHAT YOU LEARN BY COMMUNICATING WITH YOUR CHILD

If your child is suffering from chronic pain and you feel like you don't know what to do, it's time to start talking to your child. How do you maintain the balance between asking questions of your child and really listening to her? As parents, we often have difficulty just listening. We may observe our child looking forlorn and pensive. We want to ask, "What's wrong?" We want to solve the problem. (This is especially true of fathers.) If we have a child with a history of headaches or stomachaches, we may want to ask, "Are you in pain? Does your head (or stomach) hurt?" While such questions are rooted in good intentions, this approach may not be in the best interest of the child.

The problem is that once you ask your child if she is in pain, you have caused her to stop whatever she was doing at that moment and to scan her body to determine if she is in fact hurting. Once the brain puts full attention on the body and on pain specifically, the pain is immediately magnified: All the brain's perception areas become focused on the pain, and the pain is felt more intensely.

While it may be difficult, you must trust that your child will tell you if he is hurting and wants help—unless, of course, there is some underlying reason that your child feels he cannot tell you. For children with chronic pain such as headaches or belly pain, the best approach is to tell your child that you will not ask him if he is in pain, but that he is free to tell you when he is hurting and whether he wants your help.

This doesn't mean you have to let your child sit and suffer in silence when you have a good idea he is in pain. Try asking him about his day, tell him about something that happened to you that day, talk about current events, make a plan for the next day, come up with a fun game or even a chore for him to do—anything to distract him, even if just for a few minutes. The goal is to reroute the nerve impulses that are misfiring and causing the pain; the less we focus on the pain, the quicker these impulses will become weaker.

Martha's eight-year-old daughter, Andrea, developed chronic pain in her back and shoulders as well as severe headaches after an operation to remove a brain tumor. Martha learned the hard way that, for Andrea, focusing on the pain could be debilitating.

•   •   •

The best piece of advice I got that immediately showed results was not to talk to Andrea about the pain. She could really function up to a certain point, but if you asked her how she was feeling, she focused on the pain and would suddenly be aware of it again. So, as a family, we stopped asking her about it, and that immediately showed a better quality of life for her. She was still in pain, but there was an improvement right away. She was able to be more easily occupied by other things, like her computer, that were more fun than focusing on the pain. The more she was able to be distracted, the more she was able to have fun and enjoy her life.

•   •   •

Martha points out another important issue: Your child may be in pain and still become distracted or even laugh. In fact, laughing is a great tension releaser. Martha came up with other ways to help Andrea cope with pain:

- Give your child as much control as possible over her pain and her life.
- Improve your child's understanding and control by giving her information about what is wrong with her and the ways you intend to treat it in a way that she understands.
- Teach your child that what she knows, does, and feels can influence her experience of pain.
- Teach your child simple ways of coping with and reducing pain, such as distraction.

We who work with children who are in pain often ask children during the first meeting, "What do you do for your pain?" Often the response is, "Nothing works." A Canadian colleague, Carl von Baeyer, Ph.D., professor of psychology and associate member in pediatrics at the University of Saskatchewan, heard this a lot, so he began brainstorming with kids to come up with a list of things that could help:

- Taking a hot bath
- Rubbing the place that hurts
- Relaxing: "getting all floppy"
- Breathing better
- Talking to yourself about staying in charge
- Thinking about a really nice place to be
- Changing activities
- Listening to music
- Changing position
- Doing physical exercises that strengthen the part that hurts

- Listening to your body to see if it's telling you to change something
- Listening to your thoughts to see if you're stuck on a helpless, negative thought
- Telling someone about something that is giving you stress
- Paying attention to the parts of yourself that don't hurt
- Paying attention to the parts of your life that give you joy and pleasure

These are just a few ways to soothe the pain. You and your child can make up your own and post them on the refrigerator as a reminder.

HOW HER BODY REACTS

When we talk about how the body reacts to pain, we use the words *signs* and *symptoms*. Signs of pain are things the doctor notices in a patient, such as a heart murmur, an enlarged liver, or a rash. These are distinct from symptoms, which are what your child tells you he is feeling. So reported feelings of pain, nausea, or vomiting are symptoms. Pain is a stressor, and these signs and symptoms are physical manifestations of stress. The body can react to stress in a number of ways and through a number of "stress systems." These systems include the nervous system, the hormonal system, and the immune system. Each of these systems, when disrupted, can affect any organ in the body, causing multiple signs and symptoms.

When a child is experiencing pain, his body often will respond with biological signs of stress such as an increase in heart rate, blood pressure and breathing rate; temperature changes; sweating; and immune system changes. The pain can also cause symptoms such as pins and needles, muscle aches, and nausea. As a parent, you are not going to be taking blood pressures or measuring stress hormones or immune proteins. You *can* take a pulse to see if it is rapid (likely more than 90 to 100 beats per minute). One pulse point is at the wrist just below the thumb. You can also take note of other observable signs of stress such as whether your child is sweating or vomiting. You need to take into consideration what you notice physically about your child, what he is telling you, and what behavior he is exhibiting.

Together, these tell a story. It is our job, as parents, to learn the story and make sense of it. This is what I do when I evaluate a child. I notice the child's behavior, sometimes even in the waiting room. I have the nurse take vital signs (heart rate, blood pressure, height, weight, and, if the child looks ill, temperature). I also take a detailed history from the parent and child before I examine the child, which includes medical and family-related information. On the basis of the entire picture, I come up with what is called a working diagnosis, or understanding of the problem, and from there I develop a treatment plan.

Unfortunately, many of the biological signs of acute pain or stress on the body are not present in children with chronic pain. For example, more often than not, a child in chronic pain will have normal pulse and blood pressure. He will not be sweating or have changes in skin color or breathing. He may report severe pain but may not look like he is in pain; he may even be able to smile or laugh. Pain is a very subjective experience. Each child must be evaluated individually using information gathered about the patient specifically, as opposed to using a standard guide.

PARENTAL EXPECTATIONS

Parents' expectations, whether stated or not, can have a huge impact on how a child expresses his pain and even on the child's perception of pain.

Other factors that can affect a child's pain-related behavior include context and the environment (i.e., where the child is when he has the pain). For example, after Johnny was hit in the knee with a soccer ball, he played the rest of the game without any apparent change in behavior—not even a grimace. But he began to cry as soon as he got into the car after the game and complained of knee pain. Children often are reticent about reacting to pain in front of their peers but find it much easier to do so in front of parents. Thus they may hold it in until they are in a safe environment when they can let it all out. It is the same with chronic pain, even pain that the child has been living with for some time.

A couple of years ago, I was managing the postoperative pain of children who had just had surgery at UCLA. There was a 13-year-old boy who had just had major surgery and would have been expected to be pretty uncomfortable without a significant amount of pain medicine, like morphine. I had set him up with what is called a PCA, or patient-controlled analgesia device, with which he could press a button and get a preset amount of morphine delivered to him via his IV tube so that he could get what he needed to be comfortable. However, I noticed that he was not pushing his button and thus not getting any morphine. His muscles were pretty tense and his blood pressure was high, typically signs of pain, but he was denying any pain or need for pain medicine.

The intern who was working with me told me that this boy must be doing well because he did not need any morphine. I asked the intern to talk with the boy's mom outside the room while I talked with him alone. I discovered that the boy's father was in jail for selling narcotics and that his mom was worried that if her son used the morphine (a narcotic) he would become "just like his dad." Although she never told him not to push his PCA button to get morphine, he knew that it would upset her if he did and so pretended that he was fine without pain medication.

However, he clearly wasn't doing fine—his body was becoming increasingly tense, he was afraid to move, and his blood pressure was rising. Clearly he was suffering, but his concern for his mother overrode his own needs. Children are acutely aware of what their parents and other figures of authority want or expect (even if we as parents and doctors do not realize it).

TOOLS DOCTORS USE TO MEASURE PAIN

Doctors often need to quantify pain in order to prescribe the right treatment and know that it's working. To help treat children with chronic pain, a number of pain measurement tools have been developed and tested to estimate the level of pain a child experiences.

Children as young as three years of age can quantify their pain if they are offered the right tools. For children under age six, visual tools help in the understanding and explaining to others the concept of "less or more hurt." For example, we can use poker chips, pain thermometers, pain ladders, and children's faces with expressions ranging from neutral to very distressed. A child is asked to point to the number of poker chips, place on the ladder or thermometer, or face that best shows how much pain she feels. For a child who is in the hospital, frightened, upset, and in pain, asking him how he is feeling is not necessarily going to produce a reliable indication of his pain. To get the best results, it is important that whoever is conducting the test make sure the child understands that he is being asked about his hurt or "owie," not how he "feels" because his mommy is out of the room or because he is scared or hungry.

Here are some examples of pain tools:

- A vertical (up and down) line with a neutral face at the bottom (no hurt) and a sad face at the top (the worst pain possible). These lines can also include a thermometer, a ladder, or other visual items that clearly indicate the concepts of *more* and *less*.
- Lines in bright colors such as a red that become more pronounced as they move upward (as in a thermometer)
- Body drawings that the child can use to color in the part of the body that hurts, with different colors assigned as signifying a small, medium, and great amount of pain.
- Blocks with which the child builds a tower, with the number of blocks showing how much he is hurting
- The Poker Chip Scale, which quantifies the child's pain by the number of chips (0 to 4)—"pieces of hurt"—that he selects
- The Faces Scale, which shows a series of faces from happy or neutral (no pain) to very upset (the worst pain). The child is asked to choose the face that matches how he feels.

Children as young as age three years can understand the Faces Scale. Typically, older children (age 10 and up) and adolescents can use the same number rating scale that adults use. For this method, the child is asked how much pain she is in, on a scale of 0 to 10, with 0 being no pain and 10 being the most pain possible. When I asked Sammy, age 12, how much his head hurt on the number scale, he promptly told me that it was a "25!" The message he was giving me was that the pain was so bad that it was way off the scale. I got that message loud and clear!

Earlier in this chapter, I stated that the best way to approach a child's pain is by not asking him about it and therefore not focusing on the pain. Because focusing on the pain at home reduces opportunities for distraction, I typically do not ask parents to have their children keep "pain diaries" or to have their children rate their pain. I leave the rating systems for when I see the child in my office. Children seem to understand the difference between being asked about their pain in a doctor's office or hospital and having a parent ask continuously throughout the day. It is similar to having a blood test or a blood pressure assessment. Children can learn to distinguish between two types of pain care—one type that happens with the doctor and the other that happens at home.

{ CHAPTER FIVE }

Factors That Contribute to Chronic Pain

It is more important to know what type of person has a disease than what type of disease the person has.

—SIR WILLIAM OSLER (1849–1919)

Clarisse, a 12-year-old, was referred to me by a colleague. She had been in a wheelchair for several months with severe leg and back pain, as well as headaches and abdominal pain. By the time I saw her, she had undergone months of evaluations by orthopedists, rheumatologists, neurologists, and gastroenterologists, with numerous lab and x-ray tests, endoscopies, colonoscopies, and other procedures to find out what was causing the pain. After costly and lengthy testing, the specialists were stumped.

My evaluation found that most of Clarisse's pain was myofascial (musculoskeletal), which was most likely the result of sitting or lying around for too long after viral gastroenteritis that left her with ongoing belly pain (that had evolved into IBS). She also had severe anxiety and depression. The anxiety was causing her more pain. The depression was keeping her from feeling motivated enough to cope and was interfering with her sleep.

I had Clarisse begin taking an SSRI (Celexa) to help her anxiety and depression and to help her sleep. In the meantime, I prescribed a faster-acting medication (a neuroleptic) that would calm her central nervous system, because the SSRI would take about four weeks to take effect. I also recommended PT, psychotherapy, biofeedback, and Iyengar yoga. Clarisse's mom would call me daily to tell me that her daughter was still in pain. We made some adjustments to her medications, and I told her that things would not improve much until Clarisse began at least one of the nondrug therapies that I recommended.

Finally Clarisse's parents signed her up for PT, and around the same time, the medications began to take effect. Clarisse's mood improved almost immediately. She began sleeping better and exercising daily, swimming three days a week. Her mom called to tell me that Clarisse was no longer using a wheelchair. However, her mom was upset that Clarisse's belly pain had not gone away.

I wanted to say, "Clarisse is improving . . . even faster than I expected . . . she is walking, sleeping, and exercising! Aren't you excited? I am!" But I didn't. Instead, I bridled my enthusiasm, reviewed her daughter's progress with her, and told her that Clarisse was making progress and that I was sure her pain would improve. I reminded her that medication alone would not be the primary solution and that Clarisse would need to learn coping skills as well. Again, I recommended that Clarisse start psychotherapy for her anxiety and depression. Clarisse's mom was still holding out for a quick fix.

I began to realize that Clarisse's mom's reaction was related to her own anxiety about her daughter. She was especially upset about Clarisse's refusal to eat when her belly hurt; she viewed the belly pain as much more worrisome than the body pain that had kept Clarisse in a wheelchair. The more that Clarisse's mom focused on how little she was eating and pushed her to eat more, the more anxious Clarisse became about eating, and this increased anxiety produced more belly pain.

After talking with Clarisse and her mom about the food–fear of eating–anxiety–belly pain connection, I worked with Clarisse's mom on a strategy to help her daughter learn how to relax. During one appointment, I suggested to her that she needed to take care of herself, too, in order to provide a good role model for her daughter. Clarisse's mom informed me that her primary concern was her daughter and that she had no time to relax. Only after her daughter was cured would she take time for herself.

To understand chronic pain such as Clarisse's, it helps to appreciate the various factors that can create increased risk for the development of a chronic pain problem, as well as those that can magnify the pain and maintain it.

The body's pain system is dynamic—that is, it is active and constantly changing. Remember, in fact, that it is really two systems working together—pain transmission and pain control. In the transmission of pain, pain signals move from the site of the pain to the brain. In the pain-control system, the brain sends messages down the nerves to the site of the pain to turn off or reduce the pain signals. There are factors that can worsen pain by increasing pain transmission, reducing the efficiency of the pain-control system, or by increasing pain perception in the brain.

Each child needs to be individually evaluated so that as many factors as possible can be identified and treated or managed. This is in contrast to the common belief that there is one way to treat migraines, another to treat belly pain, another to treat myofascial pain (e.g., back pain, tension headaches), and it is why such simplistic treatment approaches often fail for the group of children with multiple contributing influences on their pain. (These are the children that we see in the UCLA pediatric pain clinic and who are seen at other pediatric pain clinics nationally.) These are the children with "migraines," for example, who fail to get better using the migraine medications that are typically prescribed by neurologists for pediatric migraine.

When I evaluate patients, I assess multiple factors in pain perception that are unique to each patient, including anxiety, depression, focus of attention, memory, gender, parental role models, coping ability and coping style, age and cognitive level, exposure to the pain of others, past pain experiences, expectations, perception of control, and learning disabilities.

Let's first explore the three factors that in my experience most significantly affect pain perception: arousal/anxiety, memory, and attention.

ANXIETY AND CHRONIC PAIN

The ANS is the part of the nervous system that regulates the body's homeostasis or balance. The ANS consists of two parts: the SNS and the parasympathetic nervous system (PNS). The PNS is responsible for restorative functions, like digestion. The SNS protects the body as the first response system to threat (actual or perceived threat). It readies the body for what is called the fight-or-flight response, which is activated when a person feels that she is in danger. To do this, the muscles must have enough oxygen and nutrients, so the SNS diverts blood away from the intestines and other internal organs and to the muscles. To increase the oxygen and blood flow in the muscles, the SNS causes the heart to beat faster and the breathing rate to speed up. Palms become sweaty, blood flow to muscle's increase, digestion shuts down, feelings of stress are intensified, and the body is prepared for either running away or staying put and fighting. If left unchecked, these symptoms can lead to dizziness and difficulty breathing.

Anxiety can produce these same body sensations or symptoms because it is typically accompanied by an increase in SNS activity. Also, SNS nerves connect with sensory nerves that carry information about pain and other physical symptoms to the brain. During times of anxiety, the entire nervous system can get revved up, which can cause a child to have diarrhea or constipation, as well as belly pain.

Some children are aware of their anxiety because they are aware of the thoughts and emotions that are creating the anxiety or worry. However, when sensations such as nausea, abdominal pain, or headaches come on suddenly, the child may not connect these physical symptoms to his thoughts or emotions. In this case, you and your child may see the pain as the major problem. And for the moment it is. This is because the child fears the pain, and the pain causes more anxiety, which in turn keeps the pain going. Typically, however, there is something underlying this pain–anxiety cycle.

For example, there may be something that has just happened or is about to happen (such as going to school in the morning) that is anxiety-provoking for your child. Your child may not even be aware that school makes him anxious. However, being bullied by other children, being behind in classes, or having a hidden learning disability or social problems can keep a child's nervous system generally aroused (turned on) and cause an increase in the volume of the pain signals and, therefore, more pain.

Some children have alexithymia—that is, they have a difficult time understanding what type of emotion they are experiencing. They may feel the physical symptoms of anxiety (e.g., rapid heartbeat, fast breathing, breathlessness, sweaty palms, hot/cold flashes, dizziness) but not feel anxious (or at least they do not understand what it means to "feel anxious"). The physical symptoms can be worrisome and even scary and can be accompanied by dread, and a feeling that "something bad" is going to happen.

Children also differ in their basic temperament and thus in how they respond to pain and even to symptoms of anxiety. Some children are more sensitive to pain and more reactive to it, and others have a high pain threshold. Some children notice their heart beating faster or dizziness sooner than other children do, even at the same heart rate or level of dizziness.

Further, children differ in the amount of worry that they experience. When the worry is excessive, gets in the way of functioning, and is accompanied by irrational fear and dread, the child has an anxiety disorder. One caveat, as I mentioned before, is that children with alexithymia may have many physical symptoms but not report feeling anxious, yet they may still have an anxiety disorder.

Although an anxiety disorder diagnosis is most often made on the basis of intense worry, physical symptoms almost always are present, such as fatigue, headaches, muscle tension, muscle aches, difficulty swallowing, trembling, twitching, irritability, sweating, hot flashes, dizziness, feeling out of breath, nausea, or diarrhea. Some children with milder anxiety symptoms can function well even though they are distressed by their symptoms, whereas more severe symptoms can disrupt the function of other children. Anxiety of any type will make pain worse. Below I describe the most common types of anxiety disorders (some children will have more than one type).

- **Panic disorder** is an anxiety condition in which a child feels terror that can come on with no warning. Accompanying symptoms can include heart palpitations (heart pounding and beating fast), sweating, weakness, and feeling faint or dizzy. The child's hands may tingle or feel numb, and she might feel flushed or chilled. She may have nausea or chest pain or feel that she is choking and can't breathe. She might also have fears of impending doom, feelings of loss of control, or even feelings that she is on the verge of death. Sometimes children with recurrent, episodic pain feel panic during a pain episode. The pain can bring on an actual panic attack, and the panic can bring on more pain.

- **Obsessive-compulsive disorder (OCD)** involves anxious thoughts or rituals that the child feels he can't control. He may feel the need to engage in certain rituals that he knows may not make sense but that he feels compelled to carry out, or he may be too anxious not to do them. For example, he may have to wash his hands compulsively throughout the day or check the locks on the door multiple times at night. He might feel the need to have everything even (such as touching the alarm clock three more times after he has touched it once) or to "undo" one thought with another. Some children have OCD traits that don't get in the way of their daily activities. Others have a severe version in which the whole day may be devoted to these behaviors and thoughts. For the child with OCD, there is no pleasure in carrying out these rituals or thoughts. He gets only temporary relief from the anxiety.

- **Post-Traumatic Stress Disorder (PTSD)** is a debilitating condition that may develop after a terrifying event. The event may have happened directly to the child, such as a car accident, sexual or physical abuse, or even a frightening hospitalization. Or she may have simply witnessed the event, such as seeing someone being shot or attacked. Typically she will have recurring intrusive thoughts and memories of the experience, yet may feel emotionally numb. She may have sleep problems, flashbacks where she sees the event in her mind over and over, and may avoid the activity or place where the trauma occurred. Her body may be on hyperalert so that little things can easily startle her. In PTSD, the autonomic nervous system resets itself to a lower threshold, so the sympathetic nervous system gets turned on easily, and little pains become big pains and little stresses become big stresses.

- **Social phobia**, often called **social anxiety disorder**, is characterized by anxiety and self-consciousness in everyday social situations. A child may have a persistent and intense fear of being watched and judged by others and may be embarrassed or humiliated by things she does or says. The fear may interfere with going to school and engaging in peer-related activities. Children with social anxiety often appear shy and have a difficult time making friends. They may worry way in advance of some dreaded situation, such as having to give a talk in front of the class. This condition might also interfere with going to public places such as restaurants, shopping malls, or parks. Physical symptoms can include blushing, sweating, trembling, nausea, and difficulty talking. A child may be afraid of being with people other than her family.

- **Specific phobias** are intense fears of something that poses little or no actual danger. Some of the more common specific phobias focus on closed-in places, heights, escalators, water, dogs, and injuries involving blood. Fear of clowns is a common specific phobia in children.

- **Generalized anxiety disorder (GAD)** is a condition that fills the day with exaggerated worry and tension, even though there is little or nothing to provoke it. Children with chronic pain may worry not only about their pain but also have widespread worries: their family's safety, their own safety, doing well in school even if they are getting A's. They may overhear their parents' worries about the family's finances or work and take these on as well. These worries are often accompanied by physical symptoms, especially fatigue, headaches, muscle tension, difficulty swallowing, trembling, twitching, irritability, sweating, hot flashes, dizziness, shortness of breath, or nausea. For children with pain problems, the increase in generalized anxiety-related nerve signals will further increase the pain signals anywhere in their body as well as increase other physical symptoms.

About 80% of the children who come to our pediatric pain clinic have an underlying anxiety disorder. This means that their nervous system is predisposed to being aroused, or turned on. They tend to be worriers and perfectionists and become anxious easily. Think of it as having a nervous system that is "wound a bit too tightly"—that is, their threshold for anxiety, and therefore for pain, is low. Children with anxiety disorders are more prone to developing chronic or recurrent pain. Anxiety doesn't cause the pain but it can contribute to it, maintain or feed it, and affect a child's ability to cope with it.

Therefore, for children with chronic pain, the anxiety and its underlying cause(s) need to be addressed and treated for the pain problem to resolve. If children have an anxiety disorder or are chronic worriers, even if they don't meet criteria for a diagnosable anxiety disorder, they have more difficulty coping with pain and functioning.

It is important for you to know if your child has an anxiety disorder that may be contributing to his pain. Because anxiety disorders tend to run in families, you might explore whether you or your child's other parent have symptoms of anxiety.

Treatment for anxiety can include medication (SSRIs such as Zoloft or Celexa), but medication is not always necessary. However, in cases where the symptoms are overwhelming the child, it is my experience that medication is the quickest way to calm the anxiety. Drugs also can help a child better cope with daily events that cause stress by raising the nervous system arousal set point (in a sense, like changing the thermostat on the nervous system so that it takes a bigger stressor to turn it on and create anxiety).

In the longer term, cognitive skill-building tools can reduce the thoughts and feelings that spiral into anxiety and then pain. For example, a child can be taught specific calming and mastery thoughts to replace catastrophic (out-of-control) thinking as well as breathing and other relaxation techniques. With hypnotherapy, a child can learn to use his imagination to alter anxiety and pain signals (See Chapter 9, "Individual and Family Therapy," for a discussion of anxiety and therapy.)

DEPRESSION AND PAIN

Though depression is most certainly a factor for chronic pain in children, depression typically *follows* the development of chronic pain rather than *causes* it. Pain and depression share many of the same neural pathways, the same circuitry, if you will. Serotonin is one of the neurotransmitters that ensures that the brain is healthy and functioning properly, and it is also one of the main chemicals that modulates depression. Chronic pain uses up serotonin like a car uses gas, and when the tank is empty, the car stops running. Depression occurs when the energy (fuel) of the body starts running low, and the body is not running efficiently. Brain scans reveal similar disturbances in brain chemistry in both chronic pain and depression, and some of the same medications are used by physicians to treat depression and pain.

Depression and pain problems also can develop simultaneously and be related to other factors. For example, in the article "Bullying Behavior and Associations with Psychosomatic Complaints and Depression in Victims," published in the January 2004 issue of the *Journal of Pediatrics*, 2,766 elementary school children between 9 and 12 years old who reported being bullied at school were found to have significantly more headaches, sleeping problems, abdominal pain, bed-wetting, tiredness, and depression, compared to those who identified themselves as bullies or who denied being victims of bullying.

Whether depression occurs as a result of pain or independent of pain, it can influence pain by leaving the child with little energy reserves and little motivation to be physically active or do other things that will help the pain. Depression can disrupt sleep and impair thinking and concentration, both of which can add to pain. Depressed children may cut back on daily physical and social activities, leaving them with fewer distractions and more time to focus on their pain. Their depression can spiral into feelings of loneliness, guilt, and unworthiness, with less and less ability to cope with pain, which then can become worse.

FOCUS OF ATTENTION

Think of the last time that you had a headache (or cramps if you are a woman). If you just sat and focused on it, the pain probably got worse.

The more it hurt, the more you focused on it, and the more it hurt. We know that pain perception takes place in the conscious brain. If the mind is occupied with other thoughts or planning for activities, then there is less room, so to speak, for pain-related brain activities, like pain perception.

Some children in pain have a difficult time shifting the focus of their attention. If they focus on the pain, they have a clear pathway for negative thoughts, feelings of loss of control, fear of the pain, and physical arousal that build up until they feel overwhelmed.

Distraction (filling the child's attention with other things besides pain), if only for a few seconds, can be very useful in actually reducing the pain and the negative feelings that accompany it. This is why we ask parents not to ask their child how she is feeling or if she is in pain. Such questions only pull your child's attention back to her body and her pain. The best way to reduce a pain problem is to help your child learn ways to function (such as participating in school, doing homework and chores, and engaging in physical and social activities as much as possible) even while she is in pain. If a child can function even while she is in pain, she will feel in control of the pain. Feeling in control can and will reduce your child's nervous system arousal and thus the actual amount or volume of the pain. You are not being an evil parent if you push your child to function and have expectations that he can. These are positive and important aspects of chronic pain treatment.

MEMORY AND PAIN

Each experience of our life is laid down in a neural network called a memory. This happens whether we are conscious of the event or not. For example, there is some evidence that there may be biological memories of painful circumcisions (performed without appropriate pain control), and that these memories may become reactivated during other acute pain events, such as immunizations, or that the early pain experiences may actually alter developing pain pathways.

Another example of this kind of memory is phantom pain. For example, if a person's leg is amputated after a bad accident or because of a bone tumor, the individual will have phantom sensation for about a year after the amputation. He will feel his ankles flex and his toes wiggle, and his skin may feel warm or cold, even though the leg is no longer there. This is because the areas of his brain that received signals (temperature, body position, sensation) from his leg are present and activated as if the leg were still there. If there was significant pain in the leg before amputation, the neural network that transmitted pain signals would remain active after amputation. This phantom pain can occur in the body even without the removal of a body part.

For example, I have seen many children who have had surgery that was associated with significant pain before and especially after the operation. For certain children, the pain remains even after the organ or body part has long healed. Because the memory of the pain remains in the brain, the nervous system keeps the pain going. This is one reason why acute pain needs to be well treated in all children, because there is no way to know which children will develop pain memories. In general, the more psychologically traumatic the pain-related event is, the more likely it is that the memory will be encoded (laid down) in the brain and remain as a pain memory. (For more on the role of memory in pain, see Chapter 1— "What Is Pain?" pages 27–28.)

Emotionally painful memories can also affect the way and degree to which a child experiences pain. Emotionally traumatic life experiences— such as witnessing someone being hurt or being in an accident—can be embedded in a child's memory. As a result, children may develop a lower threshold for anxiety during future events that they perceive as stressful. When this happens, what might seem to us to be no big deal may become psychologically debilitating for the child and can magnify the pain.

GENDER DIFFERENCES IN PAIN PERCEPTION

In the years I have been working with children with chronic pain, it has become clear to me that there are important gender-related differences in pain. These differences may begin to appear during adolescence, although it is unclear whether these gender differences are related to age, puberty, or other factors.

Many types of pain such as abdominal pain, headaches, fibromyalgia, and CRPS-I (RSD) are more prevalent in late-adolescent girls than in boys of the same age. This gender difference seems negligible in preadolescent children. In general, girls also demonstrate more pain behavior. For example, they may show more distress or less tolerance of pain than boys and report higher levels of pain than do boys.

There also may be psychological factors linked to sex differences that include the ways that boys and girls experience and express emotions, think, and behave. For example, in Western culture, stereotypical behaviors that are considered masculine emphasize showing that you have the ability to withstand pain (machoism), whereas being very sensitive to pain is stereotypical of femininity. Such gender role expectations can influence pain behaviors. Thus, boys' and girls' behaviors when they have pain may differ because of what they have learned are the "right" ways for boys and girls to behave when they hurt. These differences are learned rather than biological.

CHILDREN MODEL THEMSELVES
AFTER THEIR PARENTS

Children learn many things from watching their parents and from how their parents respond to them. Children learn about how to react to pain by watching how their parents react, not only to the child's pain but also to their own pain. This learning process is called modeling. Children who have parents with chronic pain who do not cope well will learn ineffective ways of coping with their own pain.

For example, if a child notices that his parent tends to stay home and curl up in a ball when she is sick or in pain, the child learns that if her own stomach hurts, the best thing to do is not to go to school but to stay home in bed and watch TV. This is the wrong message for a child to receive, for the longer children miss school, the more difficult it is for them to go back to school. School absences and catching up on missed schoolwork become added stressors that stimulate the child's nervous system and increase the severity of the pain.

Instead, parents should encourage their children to continue with daily activities even when they are in some pain. I am not suggesting that you tell your child to just "suck it up" and get on with life, but that a child who continues to do what he can when he is in pain will have less pain and get better faster. "We see many families who respond to chronic pain the way they would when a child is sick: have the child rest and take them out of all activities until they feel better," explains Dr. Lisa Scharff, a psychologist in the Pediatric Pain Management Service at Children's Hospital Boston. "When months have passed without a solution or improvement, it's time to turn a corner and try the opposite approach: The child needs to participate in activities and school before he starts feeling better. It's counterintuitive to many parents, but it works. It just takes a leap of faith and some help."

You can ensure that your child takes good care of himself by being a role model for him and taking care of yourself. Parents with children who suffer from chronic pain tend to focus all their attention on the child and forget about their own well-being. Your well-being is just as important as your child's because without you, he probably won't get better. Also, your child learns to cope in part by watching how you cope. (See Chapter 10, "Helping Your Child Cope with Chronic Pain," for strategies that you can use to help yourself help your child.)

COPING ABILITY AND STYLE

It is my experience that the way that a child copes with pain will influence the extent to which it bothers him. Active coping (doing something or thinking about something to reduce pain) is more powerful in reducing pain than passive coping (totally relying on someone else to make the pain better or simply taking medicine for the pain).

A child who is a passive coper may have a hard time at school, where he must rely on himself to get through the day. If you immediately rush to your child's aid—for example, you leave work to take her out of school in the middle of the day—you may inadvertently be reinforcing her belief that she can't cope without your help. If she feels that she can deal with the headaches or belly pain only if you are there to help her, she may try to find ways to avoid going to school out of fear of leaving you. She is also less likely to believe that she has any control over the pain, and this belief may cause her to fear it, which may result in anxiety and/or physical responses such as increased heart rate and rapid breathing, a chain reaction that can make the pain more severe.

When it comes to coping with pain, keep in mind the following:

- Children sense anxiety in their parents, and this can increase the child's own anxiety and magnify the pain.
- Pain is worse when you are paying attention to it and better if you are distracted from it. If you ask your child if she is in pain, she will scan her body looking for the pain, and find it. If she happens to be distracted from the pain at that moment, it is important for that moment to continue. It is perfectly fine for her to complain to you if she feels pain. (It is fine to ask your child about his/her day or other topics unrelated to pain.)
- Exercise is good for sleep and chronic pain. Nonimpact aerobic exercise is good for almost everyone, but especially for the child with

pain. Moderate exercise not only helps to improve the immune system but also improves the pain relief response from the brain, and it puts the body and brain in better overall health.

- Good sleep is good for pain. Impaired sleep makes it more difficult to cope with and reduce chronic pain. In addition to exercise, it is helpful to have a regular routine to regulate sleep. Your child should go to bed at roughly the same time each night, get up at the same time each day, and use the bed only for sleeping (not for doing homework or watching TV).

- Your child is improving when you see an improvement in her day-to-day functioning. For most patients, the pain goes away *after* the child is functioning normally. Dr. Eileen Yager, director of the Pediatric Pain Program at the University of New Mexico, often tells patients, "You've had this [pain] problem for months [or years], and you won't wake up and find it disappears overnight, even though we all wish it would. If you have a tiny improvement every day, that's very good."

- Methods of coping such as deep breathing, meditation, and imagery exercises can reduce pain and give children a sense of control over pain. "These are ways to put pain in the background, and to put more interesting and positive thoughts in the foreground," explains Carl von Baeyer, Ph.D., of the University of Saskatchewan. "Sometimes that means paying less attention to pain and more attention to everything else in the child's life: interests, friends, activities, goals, and plans."

AGE AND DEVELOPMENTAL LEVEL

Children learn to cope with pain through practice, and by their successes and failures. As children get older, they learn more ways to cope with pain and with other stressors such as problems at school, anxiety over not being liked, and fear about not getting better after an illness. The coping tools they use become more plentiful and diverse and, usually, more effective as they get older. As a child's mind becomes capable of more complex thoughts, his understanding of pain and how it affects him develops, and he can strategize about what to do to feel better. But in the beginning, children need help to learn effective skills.

The types of coping that younger children do when they are in pain are different from what older children and adolescents do. For example, younger children are more likely to seek comfort and physical soothing from a parent. As children age, they should be learning a greater array of self-soothing strategies and become more independent of parental assistance.

For example, they may learn that distraction can be effective and to find ways to occupy themselves with activities that take their mind off the pain. They also may learn to tell themselves that their pain will get better, not to worry, and to breathe slowly until the pain passes. Children who have difficulty coping on their own may have significant anxiety, developmental delays (e.g., they may be 15 years old but act and function at a much younger age level), or may have not learned that they have the ability to cope effectively.

LEARNING DISABILITIES

In some children, the CNS develops unevenly—that is, some parts develop more slowly than other parts, leading to a delay in specific social, motor, verbal, or other skills. A child may be extremely bright but have an uneven IQ. For example, she may score very high on either the verbal or performance part of an IQ test and relatively lower in other areas. This unevenness can create problems for a child, particularly if she is smart and motivated to do well.

There are many theories about why some children have learning disabilities; however, most of them have not been proven. Learning disabilities tend to run in families and may be inherited. Other contributors may be premature birth, early severe CNS infections, being born to a substance-abusing mother, and maternal smoking or alcohol use during pregnancy.

A bright child who tends toward perfectionism can hide her weaknesses by working harder. Learning disabilities in these children may go unrecognized until the child begins to unravel because she is no longer able to muster the energy required to continue doing well in an area where she is weak. When this occurs, her stress level may increase until her SNS becomes hyperaroused, which may cause a chronic pain condition to develop. The chronic pain problem may cause her to miss school and fall further behind, which can aggravate the pain condition by producing even more stress for her. Such is the beginning of a downward spiral of pain. Sometimes a learning disability may be so well compensated for by a child that it takes a dramatic event such as an injury to bring it to the surface.

• • •

Sophie, 11 years old, was well until a few months before coming to the pain clinic. During a competitive soccer practice, a fellow player kicked the ball, which hit Sophie in the jaw, causing a jaw injury and muscle strain. After the injury, Sophie continued to play soccer and was in a competitive game that weekend; however, thereafter she developed headaches.

Sophie's pain began behind her left ear and then spread to her neck, the left side of the face, and her forehead until she developed a hypersensitivity to even the lightest touch across her forehead, such that she needed to cut her bangs so that they would not touch her forehead. She had multiple tender points along the back of her neck and shoulders. Sophie described her headaches as throbbing, stabbing, burning, or aching, and she reported that squeezing the side of her head helped relieve the pain somewhat.

Sophie rated the pain as a range from 7 to 9 on a scale of 0 to 10, with an average of 8. She was unable to attend school or do homework at home, and spent most of her day watching TV and playing on her computer to distract herself. She stopped playing soccer and no longer talked much with her friends.

Since the headaches began, Sophie had seen her primary care physician, two neurologists, an ENT (ear, nose, and throat) specialist, an orthodontist, a chiropractor, an oral surgeon, and an acupuncturist. A small fracture of her jaw was found through dental x-rays, and she was fitted with a special bite plate to reduce strain on her jaw. Results of a CT scan of her head and jaw and MRI were all normal.

Sophie had recently started seventh grade but had had to change schools when the family moved, so this was her first year at the new school. She has always liked science best and was extremely good in math. Sophie's mother said that Sophie had always had trouble in reading and comprehension. However, Sophie had always made A's until this year, when she received two "incompletes" in social studies and language arts because she had missed so much school because of her soccer injury and headaches.

Sophie often spent hours trying to do her social studies and reading assignments. She wanted to get all A's, but she said that the work at the new school was much harder and she didn't see how she could catch up.

I diagnosed her condition as head trauma that resulted in a central headache with secondary CRPS-I of the head. She also had myofascial pain with multiple trigger points and muscle spasm. On the basis of her history, I also suspected that she had a learning disability (reading disorder) that was contributing to her headaches and pain-related disability.

Sophie had coped with, and therefore masked, the reading

disorder by being smart and a perfectionist and by putting huge amounts of time into her studies. However, the move to the new school, the stress of the difficult and increasing workload, and the school absences due to her headaches overwhelmed her. Her stress and pain mounted until she was unable to attend school at all.

Sophie was given medications aimed at CRPS (amitriptyline and Neurontin), started PT and Iyengar yoga for the muscle pain that was contributing to her headaches, and was referred for academic and cognitive testing. That testing confirmed that Sophie had a reading comprehension and written expression learning disorder. An IEP (individualized education plan) was set up through her school to provide special help in the areas where she was weak. Her school also agreed to reduce the number of written report assignments Sophie had to complete, presenting them instead as tape-recorded oral reports. Sophie was able to catch up on her work. As this happened, her headaches were reduced until she was able to return to school. Eventually, her headaches went away altogether.

•   •   •

How are learning disabilities recognized, especially in bright children? Parents need to look for relative areas of weakness. For example, a child may do well in math and science but have some problems in reading, or related skills. Even A students can have relative difficulties in one subject, such as math for instance, but the teacher may not be aware that this child is getting good grades in math only with great effort and much stress. If you suspect your child may have a learning disability, you can request that the school do cognitive and academic testing, which would include an IQ test, or you can have neuropsychological testing done privately.

Neuropsychological testing is an important tool to incorporate into any program of pain treatment in children. It can help to identify a child's strengths and weaknesses so that stress on the nervous system can be reduced. According to Dr. Leah Ellenberg, a child neuropsychologist and clinical associate professor of pediatrics at the University of Southern California's Keck School of Medicine who often evaluates our patients:

"A neuropsychological evaluation usually includes an interview with parents detailing the child's birth and development, social and emotional functioning, school history and interests, as well as family history of educational and psychological functioning. The child also will meet with the neuropsychologist for approximately six hours of individual testing, usually in two to four sessions.

"Assessment usually includes an IQ test that is multifaceted, such as the Wechsler Intelligence Scale for Children—Fourth Edition, which tests: verbal comprehension, perceptual reasoning, working memory, and processing speed. Depending on the child's age and ability level, various tests are used to assess language functioning, visual-spatial analysis, perceptual motor skills, attention, various types of memory, executive functioning, academic skills, and learning style. Other tests assess emotional, behavioral, and social functioning.

"Following testing, the neuropsychologist will meet with parents and the child to discuss the findings and recommendations. (I prefer meeting with parents alone first and then meeting with the child in the presence of one or both parents so that they can reinforce what I tell the child.) At the end of this process, parents and child should understand the child's individual issues and learning style. Particular problems can then be dealt with. For example, a learning disability may require individual tutoring or educational therapy (work with a learning specialist who can teach strategies for overcoming areas of weakness) as well as accommodations at school (extra time on tests or shortened assignments). A child with an attention problem may need a school setting with smaller classes, individual tutoring, or medication. Emotional or behavior problems may require individual or family psychotherapy."

{ CHAPTER SIX }

Pervasive Developmental Disorders

When I approach a child, he inspires in me two sentiments;
tenderness for what he is, and respect for what he may become.
—LOUIS PASTEUR

Jon, 15 years old, was perfectly healthy until two years ago, when he came down with the flu and subsequently developed severe headaches and other body pains. He has seen a pediatric ophthalmologist, a series of neurologists, and dozens of other specialists. He has had lumbar punctures, CT scans, MRI scans, and rheumatologic and endocrinology workups, all of which have produced normal results. The only medication that helps when he has severe headaches is an opioid (Vicodin), and he takes two of these tablets every day.

Jon says that his headaches are his worst pain problem and describes them as "pounding and throbbing" at his temples and under his eyes. Though the headaches are present at all times, he also has severe episodes daily, lasting from one hour to a few days. The opioid just "dulls" the pain. He rates his headaches as ranging from 2 to 10 (on a scale of 0 to 10, with 10 as worst pain possible), with an 8 on average.

Jon says he sees a psychiatrist every two to three months "for five minutes" and gets his antidepressant (Zoloft) prescription refilled. When the psychiatrist tried to increase his doses, Jon experienced shaking episodes, so the dose was reduced again. He has had trouble falling asleep, has been missing a significant amount of school because of headaches, has difficulty concentrating, and is tired all the time.

Of note, Jon was born two months premature with a low birth weight and had been a poor feeder as an infant. His speech development was delayed, and he had his own language until he was three years old. He saw a speech therapist until he was six years old. Jon's parents describe him as "clumsy." He has difficulty with both fine and gross motor skills, poor handwriting, and is unable to ride a bicycle. He had problems as a young child with separation from his mother and has had difficulty with new situations and any changes in his routine. He had an emergency appendectomy at age seven (significant pain experience or surgery during childhood can make the body more vulnerable to pain problems later), but no other medical problems.

Jon is in the ninth grade and has typically received A's, despite missing a lot of school. His father said that he expected that Jon would be a physicist one day and was upset when Jon once got a B+. Jon says that no subject at school interests him, he has no hobbies, and he does not like sports. He has never brought a friend home. He claims that he "doesn't have emotions" and admits that he has trouble expressing his feelings. Jon's mother also has had a history of headaches. Jon's father, an astrophysicist at a local university, is healthy.

The only findings on the physical examination were many tender points at the back of Jon's neck and between his shoulder blades. The only pain treatment that Jon was interested in was medication.

• • •

I diagnosed Jon's headaches as myofascial, primarily caused by chronic muscle spasm in the muscles of his head, neck, and shoulders. There were also a number of factors that likely made his headaches worse, made it difficult for Jon to cope with his headaches, and resulted in a chronic pain problem that interfered with his daily functioning.

This chapter is about developmental factors that do not necessarily *cause* pain but can increase the risk or likelihood that children will develop a chronic pain problem, can magnify it, and can make it difficult for children to cope with the pain. In Jon's case, I looked first to the fact that he had been born prematurely. Though not all children who are born prematurely have chronic pain problems, many have developmental problems. For example, some children will have subtle learning problems or an uneven IQ. This unevenness can place a strain on the CNS, and the stress can increase pain signals. In fact, Jon had many characteristics of a developmental problem called pervasive developmental disorder (PDD). PDD spectrum is the broader category in which autism spectrum disorders and Asperger's syndrome fit. Children or adolescents with PDD can have uneven cognitive, motor, and/or social development.

I began to suspect that Jon might have a PDD spectrum disorder, which in turn was causing his chronic pain problem, when I heard about his problems in verbal communication, his difficulties identifying and expressing his emotions, his social awkwardness and difficulty understanding the intentions of others, his physical clumsiness, his narrowed interests, primarily in computers, and his preference for being alone. These are all characteristics that children with PDD share on some level.

Jon also had difficulty being flexible; new situations or changes in his environment made him incredibly anxious. Jon might have been genetically predisposed to this type of neurology even without a premature birth. Jon is clearly very intelligent, even if that intelligence is not in all areas. Jon's father is also very intelligent and, like Jon, has a narrowed focus of interests, and is also somewhat shy and socially isolated. Jon's emergency appendectomy may have primed his nervous system to be more sensitive to pain signals. He said that he had flashback visions of the experience.

After our initial evaluation (conducted with our clinic's psychologist), we strongly suggested that he and his family not pursue any further medical evaluations that might actually worsen the pain by further stressing his already-sensitive nervous system. It was clear to us that medication alone would not be sufficient to treat Jon's headaches. We told him that if he wanted to feel better, he would need to reduce his chronic muscle spasm by engaging in some movement therapy of his choice, such as PT, Iyengar yoga, or both. We decided on PT (which is always one on one) as well as private yoga instruction so that Jon would get the focused attention he needed.

Jon's parents were worried that he would refuse to do the exercises. We suggested that they not nag him about doing his exercises and yoga poses. Rather, they could motivate him to do his exercises with things that were important to him. For example, he liked computer time alone just before dinner, whereas his parents preferred that this be "family time" where everyone was together reading or doing things in the family room. Jon hated that together time. His parents used that time as the motivator: For every 15 minutes of exercise and yoga practice that he did at least 4 days per week, he could earn 15 minutes of time alone on his computer during the 2 hours that had previously been family time.

Jon did his exercises. He complained the whole time, but he did them. One caveat: Never give your child new computer games or other prizes as bribes for future behavior. Such things should only be offered as rewards for your child's efforts *after* he has accomplished them, not *before*.

If you can't find a motivator strong enough to get your child to do what he needs to do to get well, you may have to let him get worse for a while, because you can't really get a child to do something if he is intent on not doing it. Your child may suffer—that is, until he can't stand it anymore. I promise that in time, he will come around and do his part to help himself get better. The hardest part of this approach is watching your child suffer. You will want to force him to take his medicine, do his exercises, or practice visualization. Whatever you decide, make sure that you and your spouse agree on a plan and stick to it. Mothers and fathers may have different approaches to helping their child. Often moms want to rescue their children whereas dads want to push their children to do more to help themselves. If your child senses this split, he will naturally take advantage of it, and even the best marital relationship will feel the strain.

Although medication was not the sole answer to Jon's pain problems, I prescribed something to reduce his CNS arousal. I chose Effexor, a mixed type of SSRI, for Jon because it is often useful for children with chronic myofascial pain with anxiety. I also suggested that he take melatonin (a synthetic version of the natural hormone our body produces) to help him sleep. I asked him to return in a month to review his progress.

He gradually began to improve, even though in the beginning he drove his parents crazy because they couldn't find anything that would motivate him. In fact, initially he got worse. I think what helped him the most were the sessions that his parents had with the psychologist to help them develop strategies to help Jon function better. In this way, his parents were able to work as a team with the support of the psychologist, who reassured them that what they were doing was proper, even though their son complained about everything they did.

They also worked out a plan with the school so that Jon could gradually increase his attendance, until he was back at school full-time and getting all A's once again. He continued to complain to his parents that his headaches were no better. However, his mood had improved; he seemed happier and was able to joke around with his parents more. He also became fully functional, which included studying for the SAT. Jon even joined a computer club and developed a group of like-minded friends, and slowly he began to feel less isolated. His parents were instructed not to ask him about his headaches (although he could complain if he wanted and they could feel sorry for him). Whenever I saw him and asked him about his headaches (especially if his parents were there), he would tell me that they were "the same." (However, he often smiled when he said it.)

Many of the children like Jon who come to chronic pain clinics like ours or others around the United States have a PDD. PDD is a diagnosis used to describe children who have a broad range of cognitive and behavioral abnormalities. What they all have in common is a deficit in social perception and interaction. Chronic pain is frequently an issue for children with PDD. Perhaps it is the combination of perseverative thoughts and behaviors (meaning that they tend to stay with one thing and not let go, or, as I tend to say, they have a "sticky nervous system") and sensitivity that results in children with PDD experiencing chronic pain more frequently than others. The most common subcategories of PDD are autism spectrum disorders (ASDs), Asperger's syndrome, and a sort of catchall category called pervasive developmental disorder not otherwise specified (PDD-NOS).

AUTISM SPECTRUM DISORDER

Autism is characterized by a delay in the acquisition of language, repetitive mannerisms and interests, strong preference for sameness in routines and rituals, lack of imaginative play and severe social difficulties, including poor eye contact and a lack of interest in others. The extent, or spectrum, of these characteristics can vary widely. Some autistic children may be extremely developmentally delayed (functioning far below age level), whereas others may be very intelligent and high functioning. As they enter the preschool years, some children with ASD begin to lose skills that they had during infancy and as toddlers. Typically, ASD is diagnosed before children with low function reach three years of age, and parents may become aware of symptoms as early as infancy.

Children with ASD tend to have more behavioral or emotional difficulties than children without this disorder. They become easily frustrated, have mood swings, and may overreact or become easily overstimulated, causing agitation, an inability to concentrate, and other maladaptive behaviors such as severe tantrums, aggression, disruptions, and self-injury.

Children with severe ASD are often difficult to communicate with, a problem that is highly distressing for the parents and children. Children who have high-functioning autism have more success communicating, but they may have trouble relating to others in a social setting or even getting through a day at school, which tends to be a much more stressful environment than home for these children.

Children with ASD may be hypersensitive to sounds, smells, touch, textures (oral or tactile) and also may have visual perception problems. For example, they may have difficulty interpreting facial expressions or understanding body language. It is interesting that a child with ASD may be hypersensitive one moment and insensitive another. This may be difficult and frustrating for parents, who may have trouble knowing when their child is really in pain. Children with ASD often are overly sensitive to commotion and crowds. This may happen because they do not filter normal sensory input and can have "sensory overload" in crowded places.

Children with ASD also have abnormal "sensory inspection and exploration." This means that in order to learn about an object, they often need to use multiple senses, such as touch, smell, even taste. It is not uncommon even for older children with ASD to put toys or other objects in their mouth, smell them, and even press the objects against their face. Some children have severely reduced muscle tone and may appear flabby or floppy. They may have difficulty picking up a raisin or other small object or putting small objects into small containers. They also tend to be clumsy and often fall or trip.

Children with ASD may engage in self-stimulatory physical behaviors such as rocking back and forth, head banging, rubbing a part of their body, or hitting themselves on the head repeatedly. It is easier to determine whether children with high-functioning autism are in pain than it is those with low-functioning autism. For the latter, the only clue may be an increase in irritable or out-of-control behavior.

ASPERGER'S SYNDROME

Asperger's syndrome is characterized by an inability to understand how to interact socially. For example, an adolescent boy with Asperger's told a psychologist that she must be having a "bad hair day" and told a nurse that she needed to lose weight. I have worked with many children with Asperger's over the years and have learned not to be offended or take personally some of the things that are said to me, because they are rarely said with bad intention.

These children have difficulties with transitions or changes and prefer sameness. They also have a great deal of difficulty reading nonverbal cues (body language) and often have difficulty determining proper body space. For example: An adolescent girl with Asperger's was avoided by her classmates at school because she would get too close to people when she talked with them.

Children with Asperger's are generally distinguished from those with high-functioning autism because autism is typically associated with marked early language delay, whereas Asperger's may not be. Although children with Asperger's may have normal language development, they may speak awkwardly, as if they were little adults. For example, one eight-year-old boy with Asperger's told me that he planned to be an investment banker and asked me (in the waiting room before our first appointment) if I had my investment portfolio in order and had I invested wisely. (I diagnosed his Asperger's on the spot.)

Other characteristics of Asperger's include clumsy and uncoordinated motor movements, limited interests, or unusual preoccupations. The mother of one boy with Asperger's told me that her son was fascinated with vacuum cleaners and that every time they went to the shopping mall, he made her stop in each store that sold vacuum cleaners so that he could inspect them.

Many of these children are highly intelligent, but they may show unevenness in their abilities. For example, they may be math or physics scholars but have significant difficulty in verbal expression, language arts, or written expression. Some show a symptom called hyperlexia, in which they learn to read at an extremely young age, almost as soon as they can talk. Many have excellent rote memory and become intensely interested in one or two subjects such as trains or sports statistics (sometimes to the exclusion of other topics). They may talk at length about a favorite subject or repeat a word or phrase many times.

Children with Asperger's often have repetitive routines or rituals and problems with nonverbal communication. Many of these children exhibit few facial expressions, and thus it is difficult for others to understand from facial cues the intentions of these children. As a result, they often have difficulty forming social relationships. A child with Asperger's may be very close to a parent (typically his mother). However, his greatest social difficulty is usually with peers. Children with Asperger's are often rule-bound and have a hard time seeing different points of view.

Whenever I diagnose a patient with Asperger's, especially a teenager who has previously been diagnosed with OCD or ADHD, I get a sense that the family is relieved to have a diagnosis and a description of symptoms that feel like they make sense. Often a patient will e-mail me after reading more about Asperger's and say "That is me, exactly!" They often feel understood for the first time.

PERVASIVE DEVELOPMENT DISORDER NOT OTHERWISE SPECIFIED

Children with PDD-NOS may not clearly fit the criteria of either autism or Asperger's syndrome but may exhibit some unusual symptoms such as social problems or focal interests. I call this "PDD-ish," which to me means that the child has some characteristics of PDD but does not necessarily show the full range of symptoms. These children often have obsessive routines and may be preoccupied with a particular subject of interest. Their need for doing things in an orderly and same manner is sometimes misdiagnosed as OCD.

Unfortunately, this kind of behavior often creates difficulty at school for the child with PDD characteristics. Depending on the severity of these characteristics, these children are seen by others as "nerds" or "geeks" or "weird" in some way. They are considered different and are often teased or avoided. They may become socially isolated but often prefer to be alone than with others (different from the child with social anxiety who feels lonely and would like to have friends but has difficulty making them). Sometimes they will team up with another "geek" who has similar characteristics and then they engage in parallel play, such as surfing the Internet together but separately, or they may play with an object like a computer or video games instead of imaginative play or some joined activity. Children who are PDD-ish often collect items such as stamps, miniature toy cars or soldiers, or Pokémon cards, although they typically do not play with these collections but just have them.

In addition to narrow interests and repetitive rituals, it is extremely common for children who are "PDD-ish" to be hypersensitive. They may hate loud noises, for example, and resist going to stimulating settings such as amusement parks. They may have an aversion to certain tastes or textures in food. For example, I had one patient who only ate beige foods, and another who only liked "crunchy" foods. They may have very sensitive skin and hate tags or seams in clothing or even being touched.

Children with PDD spectrum disorders, especially those with Asperger's, often are smart, logical, rational, and moralistic and may seem argumentative. Because they tend to stick with one thing or idea far longer than most people would and often do not let go, they often appear to be difficult.

PERVASIVE DEVELOPMENTAL DISORDER AND PAIN

Children with PDD tend to be perseverative. It is this way with the pain as well—pain comes and stays. Children with PDD are typically bright and their brains learn well, at least in some areas of learning. In fact, their brains learn so well that they also learn pain well, keeping the pain loop going and going. But because these children are smart, their brains can also unlearn the pain, or at least they can learn better ways of coping. Certain drugs may help break up the pain loop. Think of a pain loop as what happens when your child has a mosquito bite that itches. The more he scratches, the more it itches, and the more it itches, the more he scratches. You need to help your child break up the cycle with calamine lotion or Benadryl or cool water. It's the same with chronic pain.

What is interesting is that many of these children rate their pain as relatively low in intensity (a 4 or 5 on a scale of 0 to 10), yet they cannot tolerate that relatively low level of pain. This means that coping is extremely difficult for children with PDD.

In evaluating children who come to our program with PDD characteristics, I look for symptomatic areas that relate to the child's neurology, because that will tell me about her pain condition and pathways to treating it. For example, I might look for some of the following: early childhood history that included a premature or difficult birth; developmental milestones that are met early, except for language, which is often delayed; and sensitivity to certain clothing textures, or sounds, or temperature.

Because the child with PDD often has difficulty with transitions and separation from his mother, preschool or kindergarten may be difficult at least initially. Transition to middle school or high school is likewise difficult. Both of these events can cause a pain problem to begin, if it is going to. Simply transitioning from one activity (such as stopping a computer game to eat dinner) can cause a child with PDD a lot of distress.

• • •

One bright four-year-old boy named Chris who had very high functioning ASD, developed headaches after his family moved to a new house. He would curl up in a ball on his floor and cry, scream, and rock while holding his head. A pediatric neurologist diagnosed migraines and tried all of the migraine medications. However, the headaches grew worse, and Chris developed extreme side effects to all of the medications.

When I saw Chris in the pediatric pain clinic for an evaluation, I diagnosed his condition as PDD. He had a history of extreme sensitivity to clothes, touch, and sounds, and difficulty in crowded places with lots of activity, with separations from his mother, and with transitions. I also learned that the new house, besides being a new experience that he had to adjust to, was down the street from a police station and he could hear the sirens from a distance. This was so distressing for him that he began to listen for them in anticipation. Chris's entire body would shudder when he heard them.

A physical examination also indicated that he had tender points at the back of his neck and shoulders, likely related to his anxiety and to the tensing of his muscles in anticipation of the sirens. I prescribed a very low dose of Prozac, an SSRI that is often used in PDD spectrum disorders, to provide a buffer from the many external sensory stimuli in the environment and internal stimuli (his own pain sensations) that were constantly causing him distress and increasing his headache pain.

I suggested that the parents get earplugs for Chris to use whenever he wanted. I also recommended a special preschool that has experience with children with PDD and where he could learn some specific coping skills, such as how to play with other children, how to soothe himself when he was stressed, and how to go to a quiet place when he became overstimulated. Chris loved the earplugs. He soon stopped listening for the sound of the sirens and he learned to ignore the sounds until they no longer bothered him. He loved his new school that he attended three days a week for half a day, and because his parents now understood their son's illness, they became more involved and helped Chris's doctor in setting up and continuing a treatment plan.

• • •

It is often difficult for parents of children with PDD who have trouble communicating their experiences to understand how much pain their child is in. Often parents have to rely on behavior, especially changes in behavior. One patient of mine would bang his head on the floor repeatedly and scream. You may say, "Well, that is an obvious sign that the child is in pain. How could a parent not understand that?" But this was not completely unusual behavior for this child; he often yelped and screamed throughout the day. In this case, however, his behavior was unusual because he was not known to throw himself on the floor, and his screams were slightly elevated.

It is very important for children with PDD spectrum disorders to be specifically taught to modify their behaviors to cope more effectively. Although they may be most comfortable adhering to their rituals or interacting only about their specific interests, these tendencies are likely to result in social isolation just when many of these children start to actually want social contact. Many PDD children do best in environments that are highly structured, with clear rules and expectations. They can often be induced to modify their behavior with consistent, supportive redirecting.

Redirecting a child's behavior is not always as difficult as it might sound. For example, my first introduction to one 13-year-old patient was hearing him yell repeatedly, "Ow! Ow! Ow!" in the waiting room before our initial meeting. When I saw him, his mother told me that he had been doing this for the past two months since he first developed leg pain after a mild injury (he had CRPS). I suggested to him that he might want to squeeze a ball instead of yelling, "Ow!" I gave him a wad of paper towels for him to demonstrate how well he could transfer his reaction to his symptoms. To my surprise, he was easily able to do this, and he said that he felt better because he'd been embarrassed by his "ows" but didn't know how to stop.

If a child has repetitive, distressing, or annoying behavior associated with his pain, I often recommend that parents initiate a behavioral plan where the child is offered rewards or privileges for having longer and longer periods in which he does not engage in certain behavior. For example, one patient of mine had belly pain and would have spasms every two minutes where he would suddenly curl into a ball and groan loudly. This had been going on for several months and was driving his parents crazy, even though they felt bad that he was hurting. He refused to go to school because of the pain and also because he said he was embarrassed by his loud groans, over which he felt he had no control. We initiated a behavioral plan (and some medication and other interventions, such as yoga), and his parents worked out a series of incentives (rewards) for small amounts of time that he was able to go without groaning, beginning with 5-minute and then 10-minute periods, until he was able to be at school for an hour at a time without making groaning noises. He also developed a plan for himself where he learned to muffle his sounds so that they weren't so noticeable at school.

I find that giving children incentives to change behaviors works far better than restrictions and punitive actions for not doing something. The best way to motivate children is with successes. Therefore, it helps to base rewards on goals and accomplishments. Be careful not to set goals too high at first; set the initial goals so that they are likely to be successfully attained. Behavioral plans are not easy to implement, but they work well if they are used consistently. The best behavioral plans help the child to function and cope with the pain at the same time.

The following are some questions raised by the mother of a teenage patient of mine named Frank who came to us because of persistent headaches. I include these so that you can start thinking about the kinds of questions you will want to ask your child's doctor if your child has been diagnosed with a PDD-related disorder.

No migraine medications seemed to help Frank. They made him vomit, feel jumpy and nauseated, and have difficulty sleeping, and they left him with more pain. When Frank came to our program, we diagnosed Asperger's. This diagnosis helped us, Frank, and his mom understand how his neurology makes him extremely sensitive to outside stimulation and social situations as well as to medications. With this understanding, we were able to work out behavioral and medication plans that made sense for Frank's situation.

Mom: How do you know about Frank's social needs?
We can't assume that his social needs are the same as yours and mine. Though he says he is lonely at times, socializing with other peers is stressful for him. On the basis of knowledge of our other patients similar to Frank, he may have difficulty understanding or reading subtle social cues or communication. As our psychologist pointed out, "It's like being color-blind—certain information does not register. This makes it more difficult to figure out how to respond." Thus, Frank may not understand the meaning of a person's facial expression or may say inappropriate things or

may inadvertently hurt someone's feelings. Frank will need to learn certain rules to help him out socially. Further testing and training might help to sort this out, but he may always be more of a loner than others.

Mom: You mention that he is bright. How do you know?
He has a superb vocabulary. We have seen many patients like Frank, and even though Frank may be different from other kids his age, this doesn't mean that he can't be successful. Many of the great scientists and artists of history had similar neurology.

Mom: How did you know that he is bored at school?
Because all of our patients like Frank say the same thing.

Mom: How do we find out what Frank is really good at and what he should pursue besides his interest in a particular subject at school?
Testing is one way to understand his strengths. His interests are also important. It might be helpful for him to take an online career interest test: www.careerkey.org. It's free.

Mom: An alternative to a high school degree is a GED [general equivalency diploma]. Isn't there a stigma attached to listing a GED on a job application?
It is true that some employers consider a GED a lower level of achievement because many high school dropouts later take the GED test. However, if Frank obtains some college or vocational training, having a GED would probably become unimportant.

Mom: You seemed to have understood Frank before you even met him. How does his early history tell you this?
Though each child or adolescent is different, it is also interesting how alike our patients with Frank's neurology seem to be. The things that act

as clues are perfectionism, many sensory sensitivities, social avoidance (preferring to be alone), clumsiness, and the need for speech therapy early in life. These are all neurological findings that occur with a certain group of our patients.

Mom: Our goal for Frank is to be as fulfilled as possible, and we want to help him become a responsible, happy, healthy adult. What can we do?
It seems like you are already doing a great job. The path to these goals is clear: Support his strengths and abilities, and help him learn skills to cope better with his relative weaknesses.

PART III

Treating Chronic Pain

{ CHAPTER SEVEN }

Medicines for Treating Chronic Pain

On October 16, 1846, Gilbert Abbot, a Boston printer, became the first human being to go under the knife without feeling any pain. After breathing in a new chemical called ether, the man was opened up by surgeon John Collins Warren, and a tumor was removed from his jaw while he slept, as doctors and medical students looked on. After the procedure, Warren addressed his audience and declared, "We have conquered pain."

—*THE PEOPLE'S JOURNAL OF LONDON*

Unfortunately, we haven't conquered pain. Although surgery will never hurt the way it used to, pain remains.

• • •

Eleven-year-old Susie suffers from acute abdominal pain (unrelated to her menstrual cycle). Like clockwork, every two weeks she ends up in the ER with debilitating stomach pains. Each time, the doctors treat her with a morphine drip and the pain goes away (and she falls asleep), until the next bout. The doctors are stymied because their evaluations do not reveal a cause for the pain. They wonder if she is coming to the ER just to get morphine. However, Susie insists that the morphine makes her nauseated and that she would prefer that her stomachaches just go away so she doesn't have to go to the ER.

· · ·

Susie likely has IBS, a functional nerve-signaling disorder (see Chapter 3, "Chronic Pain Conditions," pages 70–77), and morphine is the wrong drug to give her. Morphine stops the brain factory from making endorphins or "natural morphine," an important component of the pain-control system. Susie was probably given morphine because her doctors didn't know how to diagnose or possibly how to treat IBS effectively. What she really needs is a better plan for pain control!

· · ·

Fifteen-year-old Michael has wound up in the ER multiple times in the past six months. He has SCD (see Chapter 2, "Diseases and Illnesses Associated with Chronic Pain," pages 37–44), which causes intense pain crises where his abnormally shaped blood cells form clots and clog small arteries, making it difficult for blood and oxygen to get to certain body parts. The ER staff at his local hospital has become increasingly unsympathetic to his pain experience; they wait longer than they should to get him medication, and then give him a lower dose of morphine than is helpful for his pain. He is sent home with an insufficient supply, and there is no plan for how to avoid ER visits and manage his pain better at home.

· · ·

In the case of Michael, the ER physicians wanted to do the right thing, but their biases about giving opioids to children, especially to a teenager, got in the way of proper treatment. They assumed that appropriate levels of pain relief would "reinforce bad behavior." However, their approach did not bring about changes in Michael's behavior. The best way to get an adolescent with chronic pain to keep asking for more pain medication or to keep coming to the ER is to undertreat his pain. If Michael had been prescribed the proper drugs to take on a daily basis and had been helped to create a plan to cope with it at home, he would have been able to reduce the pain before it got out of control. He would never have been in the ER getting opioids in the first place.

GIVING OPIOIDS TO CHILDREN

Paradoxically, many physicians use opioids for pain management in situations where this class of medications is not useful yet undermedicate when opioids are the right type of medication but higher doses are called for.

An opioid is a chemical substance that has pain-control properties and sedative effects that dull the senses and induce relaxation. It doesn't actually remove the pain, but it produces an "I know it's there but I don't care" attitude. Like many parents, doctors sometimes fear giving opioids to children because of worries about harm to young children and addiction in adolescents. When opioids are indicated as the correct medication, they should be given.

Opioid addiction, tolerance, and dependence are often confused with one another. *Tolerance* is a physiological need for more and more opioid over time. That is, the longer the child takes opioids (e.g., more than a week), the more likely that his body will acclimate to the medication and will need more to get the same effect over time. Opioid *dependence* is the withdrawal that develops if the opioid is suddenly stopped after a week or more of use. Withdrawal symptoms include sweating or rapid pulse; belly pain; increased hand tremor; insomnia; nausea or vomiting; physical agitation; anxiety; transient visual, tactile, or auditory hallucinations or illusions; and grand mal seizures. This is why a child should always be weaned from opioids—the drugs are removed gradually via lower and lower doses over time. *Addiction* is the psychological craving for a drug; that is, the individual wants it not for pain control but for some other feeling that the opioid invokes, typically for anxiety reduction. Addiction is a rare problem in children, especially in children taking drugs to treat pain.

Opioids are not the medication of choice for most chronic pain problems because opioids do not directly rebalance nerve signaling. Most chronic pain is caused by dysregulated nerve signals combined with a natural pain-control system that is not working properly. Opioids are aimed at what are called opioid receptors that normally are meant to respond to the body's natural opioids (e.g., endorphins, enkephalins), chemicals in the body's pain-control system. If these receptors are filled with opioids from outside the body (such as Vicodin), the body stops making natural opioids, resulting in a need for more and more opioids from outside. This delays the body's ability to get its own natural pain-control system up and running effectively again.

There are appropriate times for the short- and longer-term use of opioids to treat chronic pain. I do not hesitate to use opioids for certain chronic pain conditions when there is an ongoing nociceptive source of the pain, such as inflammation, pressure from a tumor, or ongoing severe active infection causing pain.

• • •

Henry was in ninth grade when he developed chronic pancreatitis (chronic inflammation in his pancreas) of unknown causes. He had severe belly pain that he described as a "knife through my back from my stomach." He was not allowed to eat for months in order to give his pancreas a rest so that it would heal. Henry received all nourishment intravenously. To allow him to attend school and not suffer, I gave him a PCA device with opioids in a little portable backpack that he could wear to school. The PCA is a computer-driven device that allowed him to deliver a set dose of morphine into his veins when he pushed a little button at the end of a tube that was attached to the syringe containing the morphine. I programmed the doses that he was allowed to give himself and the time intervals between doses. He did not give himself more than he needed to feel comfortable enough to function and feel good. When his pancreatitis improved, we were easily able to wean Henry off the opioid.

•   •   •

Below, I discuss different categories of drugs that are used effectively to treat chronic pain and describe when they should or shouldn't be used. One general caveat, from Elliot Krane, M.D., chief of the pain management program at Lucile Packard Children's Hospital at Stanford School of Medicine: "Drugs, per se, are seldom *the* answer or *the* solution. No drug works completely, and most drugs carry with them a significant price in terms of side effects. Drugs are therefore used as an adjunct, but only inasmuch as they improve function. The use of a drug that does not improve the level of function should be stopped. For example, if an opioid leads to drowsiness and depression and decreases activity, it should be discontinued even if reports of pain diminish."

OFF-LABEL DRUGS

Many of the drugs that I discuss in this chapter have *not* been approved by the U.S. Food and Drug Administration (FDA) for the treatment of pain in children. Use of drugs for something other than that for which they were originally intended is called off-label use. The FDA allows certain drugs to be sold and advertised for specific conditions for which they have been proven to be safe and effective. Once the drug is on the market, it can be used for any condition for which it seems effective. However, a drug cannot be advertised for a condition unless the manufacturer has proved to the FDA that it is safe and effective for that specific condition. Many of the drugs used for chronic pain in children, such as low doses of antidepressants, have not been approved by the FDA for pain, even though they may be highly effective.

The problem for those of us who treat chronic pediatric pain is that few pharmaceutical companies test drugs in children because it doesn't make good economic sense to do so, unless the FDA will not approve their drug unless it is tested in children. Sometimes, this lack of approval deters some doctors from using these drugs in children because they fear a lawsuit if anything happens that might in some way be attributed to the drug. However, physicians who treat children who have chronic pain will need to take these risks; otherwise, we have few medications to offer our patients.

Many of the medications that are used to treat chronic pain were originally developed to treat something else such as depression, anxiety, and/or seizures. These medications affect the neurochemical signaling in the CNS. Parents often become concerned or embarrassed when it is suggested that their child take antidepressants. However, many of the chemicals underlying depression or anxiety are the same ones that are part of the body's pain-signaling system.

If your child is prescribed one or more medications, you will probably want to find a method for keeping track of the drugs, doses, and times you are to give the drugs to your child. As your child gets older, he may want to give himself his own medication and keep track of it all himself. Though this step toward independence can be anxiety-provoking for many parents, this form of responsibility is in fact one of the many important steps for your adolescent to regain a sense of control.

Kenneth R. Goldschneider, M.D., director of the Division of Pain Management at Cincinnati Children's Hospital, says he emphasizes self-reliance and initiative in his patients. He tells children and adolescents: "The pain is not your fault, but taking care of your body is your responsibility. . . . I'm not going to nag you about taking your medicine or doing your exercises or relaxation stuff. I'll coach and I'll cheer, but not nag. Your pain will nag you, so I don't have to."

If you choose to let your older child be in charge of taking his medicines, make plans to review how your son or daughter is doing about once a week, including how much remains in the medication bottles.

ANTIDEPRESSANTS

Antidepressants raise the level of certain neurotransmitters—acetylcholine, norepinephrine, dopamine, and serotonin (chemicals that the nerve cells use to communicate with or stimulate one another)—in brain tissue. By increasing levels of these chemicals at nerve endings, antidepressants seem to strengthen the system that inhibits pain transmission. Some antidepressants may be useful in treating chronic pain because they reduce depression and improve sleep (without being habit-forming), and also because they reduce pain signals directly.

Tricyclic antidepressants (TCAs) have been typically used in the past to treat depression. Examples include amitriptyline (Elavil), nortriptyline (Pamelor), imipramine (Tofranil), desipramine (Norpramin), and doxepin (Sinequan). TCAs are used for pain control in very low (not antidepressant) doses (e.g., 10 milligrams of Elavil once at night). Sometimes just helping a child to get good sleep is enough to help the pain problem resolve. However, now low-dose TCAs are often used for abdominal pain in IBS or in some types of headaches. They are also typically used for pain that is directly neuropathic, such as in CRPS.

TCAs are nonaddictive and do not lose their effectiveness once the body becomes tolerant of them, as is the case with opioids. Unlike most anti-inflammatory drugs (like ibuprofen), TCAs do not cause stomach irritation or bleeding, and they do not interfere with the body's own natural pain-control mechanisms. Common side effects are drowsiness, constipation, dry mouth, blurred vision, weight gain, and occasionally trouble urinating.

My first choice of the TCAs for chronic pain is Elavil, 10 milligrams once at night. Elavil is the most sedating of the TCAs (other than doxepin or Mirtazapine) and thus is most useful also for promoting sleep. Though some physicians tend to use higher doses of Elavil, my experience is that if a maximum of 20 milligrams doesn't work, a higher dose is likely to bring more side effects and no further pain control. (On rare occasions, I will go up to a maximum of 50 milligrams). I also never prescribe Elavil to be taken during the day, because it causes drowsiness.

Mirtazapine (Remeron) is a TCA that increases the amount of noradrenaline and serotonin in the brain, which helps with pain relief. Though mirtazapine is often used as an antidepressant, it also is used to facilitate sleep. A major side effect is weight gain. Mirtazapine would be a good medicine to prescribe for an adolescent who has lost significant weight related to the pain problem, is not sleeping, and is also depressed. Trazodone (Desyrel) is another oral antidepressant used primarily to facilitate sleep.

SSRIs are both antidepressants and antianxiety medications but may be used for treatment of chronic pain. Those commonly used in pain treatment include sertraline (Zoloft), fluoxetine (Prozac), paroxetine (Paxil), citalopram (Celexa), and fluvoxamine (Luvox). Escitalopram (Lexapro), a newer SSRI, is reported to have fewer GI side effects than most SSRIs. Escitalopram may cause nausea or fatigue during the first two weeks of use, but these symptoms typically go away.

Venlafaxine (Effexor, Effexor-XR) is another SSRI-like drug that affects both serotonin and dopamine systems. Studies of adults with fibromyalgia have found venlafaxine to be effective in reducing pain. Venlafaxine, like most antidepressants, can cause nausea, headaches, anxiety, insomnia, drowsiness, and loss of appetite. The longer-acting form (Effexor-XR) is less likely to cause stomach upset.

Though most SSRIs have similar mechanisms of action, they all have slightly different profiles and may be prescribed for different reasons. Prozac tends to be a more activating agent (increases energy) and thus is taken in the morning and is usually prescribed if fatigue is one of the primary symptoms. For children with abdominal pain, the newer SSRIs, such as Celexa and Lexapro, tend to be used because they have a lower incidence of stomach upset than the other SSRIs. Celexa has recently been shown to be effective in children with IBS, and though not yet tested, Lexapro would be expected to work equally well.

All of the SSRI's can have side effects such as nausea and fatigue early on. Starting with a low dose and gradually increasing the dose often prevents the development of side effects. These symptoms typically go away after about two weeks at the most. Your child needs to be on the medication for about four weeks before you can typically begin to see changes. You will typically notice changes before your child does. But it's best not to say anything until your child also notices the changes for herself. Some of the medications, like Zoloft, which are used to reduce depression or anxiety, can interfere with sleep in some children (in which case your child should take it in the morning with breakfast) or cause sedation (in which case your child should take it at night).

How antidepressants and SSRIs work to affect pain directly is unknown. However, I like to think of them as giving boosts to the body's natural pain-control system so that it will work more efficiently and effectively.

Some children with the neurology for anxiety disorders or who have a tendency to be worriers and perfectionists are at risk for the development of chronic pain. We know that when children are anxious, their nervous system gets revved up, increasing the magnitude of their pain signals. SSRIs and related drugs can reduce anxiety and help lower the volume on pain signals to the brain. This category of medications also works directly on the emotional brain and can quiet fear centers and other reactive parts of the emotional brain. These medications act as a buffer to allow the child to learn other tools to reduce pain and anxiety, so that eventually he will not have to take the drug at all.

• • •

Ten-year-old Cindy had fibromyalgia and problems sleeping. She was taking Elavil when I first met her, but it left her drowsy in the morning, even if she took it earlier in the evening. After months of sleep deprivation and chronic pain, Cindy's mood appeared depressed and she seemed sad, even though she denied this. Her parents said that she had lost interest in all of her favorite activities and was often tearful. Rather than prescribe a specific medication for sleep, I decided to treat her with an SSRI (Zoloft) and see if the sleep problem was primarily related to her depression. Also, I knew that inadequate restorative sleep could be perpetuating the fibromyalgia. After a month, when I saw her next, her mood seemed markedly improved and her parents reported that they had their "old Cindy" back. She was also sleeping better, her function was improved, and she was doing PT and hypnotherapy.

ANTIANXIETY MEDICATIONS

Drugs called beta-blockers are typically used for people with heart problems, because they relieve stress on the heart by slowing the rate at which the heart beats. They have also been used to treat anxiety associated with many bodily symptoms, such as palpitations (anxiety-associated rapid heartbeats). When people are anxious, such as during a panic attack, the SNS becomes active and produces a number of anxiety-related physical symptoms such as palpitations, sweaty palms, or rapid breathing. By blocking the action of these sympathetic nerves, beta-blockers reduce these anxiety-related symptoms and help calm the child.

Beta-blockers have also been used for many years to prevent migraine headaches. Whether beta-blockers work on pain systems directly or indirectly through reduced anxiety and arousal is unknown. However, they can be very effective in reducing pain. The most commonly used beta-blocker is propranolol (e.g., Inderal).

* * *

> Steven is a 15-year-old with a history of SLE, an autoimmune disease that can be associated with pain. After a lengthy hospitalization because of severe headaches, Steven was discharged with no clear diagnosis for his headaches.
>
> He was extremely anxious despite the high doses of an SSRI (Prozac) that his rheumatologist had prescribed three months earlier. He was quick to become anxious over even small changes in his breathing or heart rate and began focusing on his body. He told me that his face flushed readily and this scared him and that he was extremely sweaty all the time and thus always thought he had a fever. I diagnosed tension headaches and panic over his illness.
>
> I prescribed propranolol because his SNS seemed turned on, which I thought was aggravating his headaches and maintaining his anxiety symptoms. With high enough doses (he eventually was taking 50 milligrams three times a day), his heart palpitations and constant sweatiness improved, his headaches got better, and he stopped focusing on his body and was able to engage with friends and return to school.

* * *

Benzodiazepines are another type of antianxiety medication. I rarely use them for children with chronic pain. Only occasionally when I have a patient who has panic attacks will I prescribe them, and only early on until an SSRI and behavioral therapy work to control the anxiety. Examples of benzodiazepines include lorazepam (Ativan), diazepam (Valium), alprazolam (Xanax), clonazepam (Klonopin), flurazepam (Dalmane), triazolam (Halcion), temazepam (Restoril), and others. The most commonly used of the benzodiazepines in children with chronic pain and concomitant anxiety disorders are Ativan or Klonopin. Benzodiazepines do not work on pain signals but rather help pain indirectly by reducing anxiety.

Benzodiazepines are typically not good medications to use for sleep because they block restorative sleep, the type that is helpful in reducing pain. Common side effects of benzodiazepines include sedation and dizziness, among others. They are also habit-forming and should not be stopped abruptly, because withdrawal could occur.

NEUROLEPTICS

Neuroleptics are a group of medications that are often used to treat severe anxiety, nausea and vomiting, or psychosis. Thioridazine (Melleril) may be useful for children with IBS who have nausea and/or recurrent bouts of abdominal pain. Besides reducing nausea, this medication also rapidly reduces arousal in the CNS, which in turn can reduce acute bouts of pain not only in children with IBS but also in other chronic pain disorders. Mellaril can be especially helpful during an acute pain episode.

Chlorpromazine (Thorazine), a stronger antianxiety medication in this category, can be helpful for children with chronic pain who also have major CNS arousal. Prochlorperazine (Compazine) is probably the most commonly used of this class of drugs for nausea and vomiting but also has the most side effects, including shakiness, the need for constant movement, and torticollis (where the head moves back in spasm). Benadryl is an effective, fast treatment of these side effects. There are few side effects with low doses of Mellaril or Thorazine except for sleepiness, although in high doses these medications can cause dizziness related to a drop in blood pressure. An electrocardiogram (ECG or EKG) should be reviewed before starting Mellaril.

Risperidone (Risperdal) is another neuroleptic that acts by blocking subtypes of the neurotransmitters dopamine and serotonin. It is used often in children with tics or Tourette's syndrome and as an antipsychotic drug. For children who have a neurology associated with tics, ASD, Asperger's syndrome, or other PDDs and have chronic pain, risperidone can be very effective in reducing pain.

• • •

> Sandy is a 14-year-old with a three-year history of severe hypersensitivity to sound, touch, and smells and with total head pain. She wore two pairs of very dark sunglasses even indoors, was in a wheelchair because changes in position and standing caused head pain, and wore a kerchief to protect her head. What also bothered Sandy (and even more so everyone around her) was a long-standing, chronic, loud, barking cough. She had been evaluated for the cough by pulmonologists, allergists, and head and neck surgeons, and no one could find the cause.
>
> After a prolonged outpatient treatment program, she was admitted to our eight-week intensive inpatient pain rehabilitation program. During that time, we helped Sandy's mother implement a behavioral plan to help Sandy become more functional. Sandy worked with a psychologist to learn coping skills and also was given both an SSRI (Effexor-XR) and a low dose of risperidone for her cough, which we believed to be a tic. By the time she left the hospital, she was wearing only a light pair of sunglasses, was out of her wheelchair, was able to engage with other teenagers, no longer wore her kerchief, and no longer had a cough.

ANTICONVULSANTS

Anticonvulsants are drugs that reduce CNS irritability. While most anticonvulsants typically are used to reduce or prevent seizures, they can also be helpful for chronic pain, especially neuropathic types of pain related to nerve hyperexcitability, such as CRPS.

The most common anticonvulsant with the least side effects that is used in treating pain is gabapentin (Neurontin). It may cause drowsiness but often has minimal to no side effects when used appropriately. In children, doses start relatively low and increase until symptom relief is achieved. For example, a typical starting dose might be 100 milligrams three times a day. I will then increase the doses by 100 milligrams per dose every one to two days, up to a maximum of 600 milligrams three times daily, and then I tend to spread the medication to four times daily, up to a maximum of 900 milligrams four times a day. Sometimes Neurontin can be given at night to enhance restorative sleep. I tend not to use the anticonvulsant Topamax because it tends to reduce memory and learning; other options include Trileptal Keppra.

MUSCLE RELAXANTS

There are a number of medications that relax skeletal muscles, such as those in the back and neck. These drugs may be helpful in myofascial (musculoskeletal) types of pain, such as low back pain, tension headaches, or other pain related to muscle spasms. The common drugs in this category include cyclobenzaprine (Flexeril), metaxalone (Skelaxin), methocarbamol (Robaxin), tizanidine hydrochloride (Zanaflex), and baclofen. The common side effect is sleepiness. Typically, PT or Iyengar yoga can be much more effective for myofascial pain than muscle relaxants, so I tend to use the latter sparingly.

TOPICAL AGENTS

Topical anesthetics (e.g., Lidoderm patches) may have a role in the treatment of chronic pain, although this has not yet been proven—there are no studies in children for this purpose. (There are some topical creams used for numbing the skin for needle sticks.) The 5% lidocaine patch (Lidoderm) is the only topical anesthetic agent to receive FDA approval for the treatment of neuropathic pain, such as CRPS-I. The patches can also be helpful in some children when applied over tender spots in myofascial pain or in fibromyalgia. Patches can be applied for up to 12 hours (the patches must then be removed for 12 hours). Side effects of topical anesthetics are minimal and include skin irritation and swelling, which usually disappear within two to three hours after the anesthetic is removed from the skin.

OVER-THE-COUNTER OR NONPRESCRIPTION ANALGESICS

Over-the-counter (OTC) analgesics may be the most widely used and least understood of the medications available for people with chronic pain. This class of drugs includes aspirin, acetaminophen (Tylenol), naproxen sodium (Aleve), ketoprofen (Actron, Orudis KT), and ibuprofen (Advil).

Aspirin, ibuprofen, naproxen, and ketoprofen belong to a subgroup known as NSAIDs. They reduce inflammation caused by arthritis, connective tissue disease, and injury by blocking prostaglandins, a chemical involved in pain signaling. These drugs reduce adhesiveness or stickiness of platelets (a factor in the blood involved in blood clotting). Thus they should not be used for treating pain in children who also have a bleeding disorder, such as hemophilia, or in those who might have low levels of platelets, such as in children with leukemia or during the acute phase of mononucleosis or other viral illnesses.

OTC medications such as the ones mentioned here can be very helpful in reducing relatively low levels of pain in a child who suffers from recurrent myofascial pain, migraines or daily muscle tension headaches, or recurrent menstrual cramps. Because they may cause GI upset or even bleeding, they should be used with caution and should not be taken on an empty stomach.

Acetaminophen (Tylenol) does not have the same effects on platelets or on the GI system that NSAIDs do. However, though it is a mild analgesic, it also does not have the same effects on inflammation that NSAIDs do. Tylenol can be toxic to the liver, so it is important to give only the dose recommended on the label. Some medications, such as Vicodin or Percocet, are combination drugs that include acetaminophen and can also damage the liver if too many are taken in a day. These combination opioids and acetaminophen are prescription only, and you should check with your child's doctor about the total amount in a day that is safe for your child to take. Some NSAIDs, such as Bextra (valdecoxib), are available through prescription only.

When using OTC drugs, be aware that the brand name tells you about the manufacturer, not about the medicine. For example, Tylenol PM is in no way the same thing as Tylenol. It is important to read the medication ingredients to know what you are giving to your child, including the dose of the medication. Some newer types of NSAIDs called COX-2 (cyclooxygenase-2) inhibitors (e.g., Celebrex) are available only by prescription and, although not well studied in children, can be useful in some cases.

•   •   •

There are three chapters in this section of the book, each of which covers a specific aspect of an overall treatment plan for chronic pain. You have just finished reading the first of these chapters. In the following two chapters, we will discuss complementary therapies and psychotherapy. In most cases, a treatment program includes more than one of these aspects, and typically, the program uses all three. When patients are referred to me by other doctors because they have been unable to treat the child's pain, I almost always find that the only approach used has been pharmacological. In my experience, only the most straightforward pain problems can be treated solely with drugs or surgery.

It is crucial for parents—and a child if he is old enough—to understand that the goal of treatment is to help the child's body begin to function normally as it did before the pain occurred. To this end, the various treatments, both drug and nondrug, are aimed at restoring balance and homeostasis in the body and reversing the cycle of pain.

A key component in the healing process is the expectation that the pain will get better. Quick solutions don't usually work for chronic pain problems. Children who do the best over time make slow and steady progress in functioning first. If a child has been in pain for a long time, it will likely take close to that amount of time for the pain to resolve.

{ CHAPTER EIGHT }

Complementary and
Alternative Therapies

*The greatest mistake in the treatment of diseases is that there are
physicians for the body and physicians for the soul,
although the two cannot be separated.*

—PLATO

Jack is a five-year-old who has had chronic headaches since
the age of four. Typically, he gets one every other day. When
they occur, he cries continually and is usually inconsolable, demanding more and more attention from his mother. Jack was
found to have childhood migraines. Medications provided by the
neurologist gave intolerable side effects with no relief. Recently,
however, Jack's mother has learned a series of relaxation and imagery techniques, which she and Jack practice together. When
the pain first starts, Jack and his mom lie down together and be-

gin by taking long, deep breaths. Jack's mom urges him to relax and think about something he likes to do such as playing on a swing in the park. Jack's mom begins by describing the sights, sounds, and feelings of the park and then asks Jack to describe them and also to notice how comfortable and relaxed he is feeling as he continues to breathe deeply. After several weeks of practice, Jack is able to relieve much of the pain. He has also discovered that he can sometimes stop the headaches on his own when his mom is not around.

•   •   •

Often we discount what is new to us or what we don't understand. But many nondrug options have been found to be highly effective in the treatment of chronic pain in children. As many nontraditional therapies have come into popular use, and as the public has become dissatisfied with the conventional medical approach to many conditions such as chronic pain, more research is being done to test the effectiveness of these therapies. Many nontraditional therapies have become so popular today that the U.S. Department of Health's National Institutes of Health established the National Center for Complementary and Alternative Medicine (NCCAM) to oversee the funding and selection of research to be funded in this area.

Complementary and alternative medicine (CAM) is described by NCCAM as "a group of diverse medical and health care systems, practices, and products that are not presently considered to be part of conventional medicine." *Conventional medicine* in this context is defined as "medicine as practiced by holders of M.D. (medical doctor) or D.O. (doctor of osteopathy) degrees and by their allied health professionals, such as physical therapists, psychologists, and registered nurses" (see: http://nccam.nih.gov/health/whatiscam/).

As I mentioned in Chapter 7 ("Medicines for Treating Chronic Pain"), in treating pediatric pain we must rely on many treatments that have not been studied in children; otherwise, we would have very little to offer in the way of drugs or other treatment. This does not mean that many of the therapies are not safe and effective—they most certainly are.

However, there are areas that fall under the umbrella of CAM that concern me; this includes the use of megavitamins, herbs, and other botanicals. Even though they are "natural," these are still potent substances and could have an impact on a child's developing organs. Herbal remedies also may interfere with the metabolism of prescribed medications or interact with these drugs to create a toxic effect. When deciding to use herbs and botanicals, it is important to review with the prescribing clinician the other medications that your child is taking and to ensure that there are no toxic drug reactions or potentially harmful effects of the herb. I also worry about invasive procedures such as high colonics and other remedies that claim to remove toxins in children, because such procedures could potentially sensitize already sensitive nervous systems in children with chronic pain, as well as remove needed nutrients and salts.

Beware of exaggerated claims about so-called natural drugs and therapies, especially those on the Internet. Also, personal stories of medicines or therapies that "worked wonders" for relatives or for the friend of the neighbor down the street may not be the right treatment for your child, even if he seems to "have the same pain problem." First, what *seems* like the same thing may not be. Second, even pain problems that bear the same name may represent different conditions in adults and in children. For example, fibromyalgia in adults is different from juvenile fibromyalgia. Use your best judgment and talk to your child's doctor about any concerns you might have. (Remember that talking with *your* doctor is different from talking with *your child's* doctor, unless you and your child have the same family medicine physician.)

When you decide on a CAM therapy, regardless of the type, interview the clinician first. (Conversely, if the practitioner doesn't ask you or your child any questions and plunges into treatment, I would be wary.) I think it is important for a parent to ask questions such as the following:

- What is your training in this therapy?
- How long have you been practicing?
- Have you worked with children before? If so, for what conditions?
- What benefits can be expected from this therapy in general and given my child's particular pain problem?
- How long before I can expect to see benefits, and how often do children need to come before benefits can be seen, on average?
- What are the risks and side effects, if any?
- Will the therapy interfere with conventional treatment?
- Will the therapy be covered by insurance?
- Are you willing to review your plans and the treatment with my child's physician?

I view chronic pain from a mind–body perspective. This is why I use and recommend the integration of CAM with more traditional psychological and pharmacological therapies for children with chronic pain. In our pediatric pain program at UCLA, we incorporate various CAM therapies in an integrative way; we all communicate with one another about patients. Our team consists of an acupuncturist and Chinese herbalist, biofeedback therapist, physical therapists with expertise in chronic pain, hypnotherapist, Iyengar yoga teacher, massage therapist, art therapist, energy therapists, craniosacral therapist, a meditation teacher, and a medical psychologist as well as psychology and child psychiatry trainees and medical students.

Many of the CAM therapies come from ancient healing arts that date back many centuries. And they have the same goal: to restore balance and harmony within the body and mind (and spirit for some). In a somewhat different way, this is also the goal of Western medicine: to restore homeostasis or balance to the bodily functions. For this chapter, I asked our CAM practitioners to help me to talk about their chosen therapy, how they work, how to decide which CAM therapy is right for your child, and some tips for finding the appropriate practitioner.

ACUPUNCTURE

Many CAM practitioners believe an energy force flows through the body. You can't see this energy, but if its flow is blocked or unbalanced, you can become sick. Different traditions call this energy by different names, such as *Qi* (pronounced "chi"), *prana*, and *life force*. Unblocking or rebalancing your energy force is the goal of these therapies, and each one accomplishes that differently. Acupuncture, for example, is intended to restore natural energy (Qi) through the insertion of needles into points along energy pathways (meridians) in the body. The needles help stimulate the energy flow.

Acupuncture has been used effectively to treat headache pain, menstrual cramps, tennis elbow, fibromyalgia, myofascial pain, osteoarthritis, low back pain, carpal tunnel syndrome, and nausea and vomiting related to chemotherapy.

Our UCLA pediatric pain program acupuncturist, Michael Waterhouse, M.A., L.Ac., studied in Japan and helped us to establish this important part of our program. As part of our pain team, Mike not only understands acupuncture and Chinese herbs but also understands chronic pain and child development. Above all, an acupuncturist must relate well to children and be able to communicate with parents how the treatment works and the goals of treatment. I asked Mike to explain how acupuncture works:

"Acupuncture is the insertion of fine needles into the body at specific points and has been shown effective in the treatment of specific health problems. These points have been mapped by the Chinese over a period of two thousand years. Recently, electromagnetic research has confirmed their locations. How deep the needles go depends upon the nature of the problem; the location of the points selected; the patient's size, age, health; and the acupuncturist's style or training. Usually, needles are inserted into the skin from one quarter to one inch deep. Acupuncturists should use sterilized, individually packaged, disposable needles. Needles should not be saved and reused for later treatments. The patient should feel some light cramping, heaviness, distention, tingling, or electric sensation either around the needle or traveling up or down the affected meridian, or energy pathway.

"Modern Western medicine cannot explain how acupuncture works. According to ancient theory, acupuncture allows Qi to flow to areas where it is deficient and away from where it is excessive. In this way, acupuncture regulates and restores the harmonious energetic balance of the body. And, according to this practice, it is disharmony that is said to cause disease.

"While acupuncture involves the technique of inserting tiny threadlike needles along meridian lines of the body, its complex system of diagnostic methods takes into consideration the person as a whole, not just isolated symptoms. Acupuncture treats and strengthens the physical condition and controls pain. The aim, as practiced in Asian medicine, is not necessarily to eliminate or alleviate symptoms. The objective, rather, is to increase both the ability to function and the quality of life."

Acupuncture is not usually thought of as a primary option for relieving pain in children and adolescents. One theory holds that because acupuncture treatment most often involves the use of needles, and because most children are afraid of needles, they would be unwilling to undergo (and their parents would not want to subject their children to) a form of care that involves needling. In my experience, this is not the case. I have found that most children are accepting of acupuncture. However, this acceptance depends heavily upon the acupuncturist's ability to relate to children.

• • •

Eight-year-old Richard liked the "sleepy" feeling that he would get after each acupuncture session. He said that in the beginning, he was a little afraid of the needles because it always hurt when he had needles at the doctor's office. But he said that "Dr. Michael" let him hold one and even put it into his arm and that it felt "weird" but didn't hurt. He said that he would sometimes get a little "buzz" when the needles first went into his body but that that went away and he felt calm and relaxed, ". . . kinda like I was sleeping or dreaming, but not quite." Richard said that being in our acupuncture research study and having "Dr. Samantha" talk with him and remind him to imagine being in his favorite place together with the feel of the needles was the "best feeling of all." He said that he "really, really got relaxed" with both of those things together.

• • •

The number of treatments needed depends on the duration, severity, and nature of your child's complaint. There may be a release of endorphins after an acupuncture treatment. The release of these morphinelike substances can make some children feel excited and energized but others feel relaxed, calm, and even sleepy.

Acupuncture practitioners are licensed and regulated health care professionals in about half the states in the United States. In states that do not currently require licensing, patients should ask their practitioner if he or she is certified by the National Certification Commission for Acupuncture and Oriental Medicine. Acupuncturists who have passed this exam are entitled to add *Dipl. Ac.* (diplomat of acupuncture) after their name.

Not all the acupuncture practitioners provide service for children. Finding the right medical acupuncture provider for your child is no different from finding a good pediatrician. For a referral to a trained physician acupuncturist, contact the American Academy of Medical Acupuncture. Its members are all licensed doctors of various medical specialties, and they have more than 200 hours of special training. There are a wide variety of ways to find an acupuncturist. You can try www.medicalacupuncture. org. Alternatively, go to the medical board Web site for your state. It should have a list of licensed acupuncturists. You can also ask a pediatric pain specialist to recommend a practitioner for your child. (See Appendix B "Pediatric Pain and Gastrointestinal Pain Programs.")

BIOFEEDBACK

Biofeedback uses a computer or other feedback device to assist your child in managing symptoms by becoming aware of and learning to voluntarily control physiological changes associated with the stress response. These monitored changes may include muscle tension, skin temperature, sweat gland response, brain wave activity, or breathing rate.

During a biofeedback session, a trained therapist applies electrodes or other sensors to various parts of your child's body. The electrodes are attached to devices that monitor your child's responses and give him visual and/or auditory feedback. For example, he might hear tones and see colorful graphs on a monitor that display changes in his muscle tension or skin temperature. With this feedback, he can learn how to produce voluntary changes in body functions, such as lowering muscle tension and sweat gland response or raising skin temperature. These are signs of relaxation. The biofeedback therapist also will teach your child different relaxation skills such as breathing, muscle relaxation techniques, and imagery.

I asked Colleen Werner, R.N., a nurse who was our pain program biofeedback clinician for many years, to talk about her personal perspectives on the use of biofeedback with children with chronic pain:

"Biofeedback is a method of monitoring changes in the nervous system. I use three types of feedback monitoring: muscle tension, hand temperature, and sweat gland response. Each measurement changes in response to higher and lower levels of tension. For example, with biofeedback monitoring, a child can see and feel how tense or relaxed her muscles actually are. Once she is aware of these levels, the child can learn ways to change them.

"The point of using biofeedback for chronic pain management is to help children learn to be aware of how their body reacts to different experiences and also to gain physiologic control of the branch of the nervous system that is always activated by pain or stress. Everyone who has ever been in pain knows that the more pain you have, the more stress you feel. And the more stress you feel, the more pain you have. So, through biofeedback, we attempt to break the stress–pain cycle. Usually there are quick changes, but even if at first there is little change in the pain itself, as the child gains more control over his body, the pain experience also becomes more manageable.

"Self-empowerment is the ultimate goal of biofeedback training. A child uses the training and equipment to gain skills in body awareness and response control. As he develops his skills, his symptoms may lessen or disappear, he will increase his energy and confidence, and he may be able to stop using medications. There are many practical methods of applying his new skills in everyday situations. A simple example is to use deep breathing before a test. A more complex example is having kids go into a stressful situation while they are being monitored with biofeedback instruments. I might take a child who is anxious in crowds to a mall and have him monitor himself in response to being around large numbers of people. Initially it might be hard for the child to relax, but eventually, using biofeedback skills, he can relax and be comfortable in that situation. It is a method of stress desensitizing.

"Habits of tension take some efforts to undo. Pain is a signal of wear and tear. If the stress response has been on high for a period of time, it can often manifest itself as pain. The point of biofeedback training is to have people learn that they have the ability to change habits of tension and learn about new strategies in pain management.

"Some children are resistant to the notion that they can control their pain. Usually it is because they are so used to not having control. In some cases [pain] can actually serve children in meeting their needs. I remember specifically one girl with migraines. She really used her headaches as a way to get out of doing things she did not want to do. She was afraid that if she didn't have migraines, she would have to say no and there would be all sorts of problems. Once she understood that she was in control of her migraines, I said I would just show her how to get rid of them, but she didn't have to if she didn't want to. While she enjoyed having some choice about experiencing her pain, there was important work to be done in helping her to develop more effective ways of meeting her needs. One purpose of treatment is to develop healthy alternative ways of dealing with the needs that pain sometimes fills. I am always looking for ways to empower people. Giving them a choice about their pain makes all the difference.

"Biofeedback is a fun and painless way for children to learn body awareness, relaxation, and pain and stress management skills that they will be able to use throughout their lives. As with any educational challenge, both timing and motivation matter. If the timing is right and motivation high, changes can occur during the first session and most definitely by the fourth. If no changes are noted after a month of treatment, I will usually stop treatment and suggest alternatives. I generally see kids once a week for a three-month period of time."

There is no license for biofeedback. Most practitioners have other licenses, such as R.N. (registered nurse) or MFT (marriage and family therapist), or are physical therapists. There is, however, biofeedback certification. Most states have their own certification process, and there is national certification as well. To find a biofeedback therapist, contact your state biofeedback society and ask for practitioners with certification and specialization in pediatric pain.

THERAPEUTIC YOGA

There are many different forms of yoga being taught today. In our program, we use a type of yoga called Iyengar yoga because it is highly therapeutic and safe for people with medical conditions, including chronic pain. In therapeutic yoga, the yoga series is matched to the health care needs of the child and changes as the child progresses. The yoga poses are intended to correct health-related problems, both in body structure and in internal organ function. Iyengar yoga teachers must have a minimum of five years of training before they are certified. It is important that a yoga exercise program is developed by someone who knows human physiology and can tailor the yoga program to the needs of the child with chronic pain. For this reason, I suggest private lessons rather than group classes until the child is familiar with the poses and can easily do them on his own.

Beth Sternlieb is the certified therapeutic Iyengar yoga teacher in our program. I have asked Beth to talk about Iyengar yoga:

"Iyengar yoga is a traditional form of yoga based on the teaching of the Indian master B.K.S. Iyengar. His method of teaching is orderly and progressive, and the postures are adjusted to meet the physical conditions and needs of each student. B.K.S. Iyengar developed a method of teaching that enhances the therapeutic benefits of yoga and a way of doing yoga postures and breathing that could be adapted to students of all ages, levels of experience, and ability. His method brings awareness, circulation, strength, and flexibility to various parts of the body to maintain optimal health.

"Iyengar yoga stresses precision and correct alignment in all postures and makes use of props, such as wooden blocks, belts, and blankets. With the aid of props, students who are stiff, weak, or unable to hold a yoga pose for the necessary amount of time can use physical support to get the desired result. A well-trained, experienced teacher can use props to address health problems. For example, lying in a backbend over a chair stimulates the adrenal glands; doing standing poses, like Trikonasana (Triangle Pose) against a wall, can teach correct alignment and relieve pressure on the lower back.

"Adrienne, a 10-year-old girl with severe abdominal pain, came to me to learn yoga to help with debilitating pain that was a result of many complications following abdominal surgery. She had developed the habit of gripping her abdomen in pain and in anticipation of pain. As she lay over blankets and pillows in passive backbends and named these poses herself (e.g., comfy pose, puppy pose), Adrienne learned to release, relax, and let go of abdominal tension. She began to understand how guarded she was and how vulnerable she felt when her belly was open and exposed. Over time, she learned to tolerate more sensation there without instinctively gripping and guarding herself.

"I use Iyengar yoga to help children, adolescents, and young adults with a variety of chronic pain problems. The combination of medical care, yoga practice, and other therapies as needed, including psychological counseling, helps many children to overcome their obstacles to live full and productive lives. Kids with chronic pain problems have been betrayed by their bodies. At a time when they should be gaining more and more independence, they are having their confidence and autonomy undermined. One of the most important things that Iyengar yoga offers these kids is a feeling of mastery. Through their own skill and actions, they can take charge of their healing and solve their chronic pain problem by virtue of their own effort.

"Jenna, a young woman in her early twenties, came to study with me after being diagnosed with rheumatoid arthritis. Depressed and frightened by the prospect of living with a chronic, debilitating, and painful disease, she came to the UCLA pediatric pain program looking for strategies that could improve her health. She decided, along with taking the medications recommended by her rheumatologist, to try yoga.

"In the months leading up to her diagnosis, Jenna's quality of life had deteriorated rapidly. In September she was healthy and active, playing volleyball, hiking, and Rollerblading. By April, the smallest movements were painful. She walked slowly with a limp, it hurt to roll over in bed, and she needed help to brush her hair. Jenna experienced pain, tenderness, and/or swelling in almost every joint in her body—feet, knees, hips, shoulders, elbows, wrists, fingers, neck, and jaw. I wanted her to know that no matter how bad it got, there was something we could do that would help. We might not make the problem go away completely, but we could give her some relief.

"We began with mostly passive inversions and passive backbends. She hung upside down on ropes and lay over chairs and bolsters. The inversions would help her immune system and the backbends would lift her mood. Eventually I taught her certain poses, like handstand, to give her a feeling of confidence and optimism. Even for students without health problems, there is something unbelievably exhilarating about kicking up into a handstand. When Jenna kicked into a handstand, she used a slant board under her hand because of the problems she had in her wrists. She found that the pose actually made her wrists feel better and improved her range of motion. Soon she was doing standing poses with a quarter round [a wooden block that is a quarter of a circle and is used to ensure proper alignment in the leg] under her foot to help with the pain in her feet, ankles, and knees. If something in particular was causing her pain, I made sure to address it in class with specific poses that brought relief. I also encouraged her to practice on her own at home as she needed to.

"Over the next several months, Jenna's health improved rapidly. By fall, she was walking normally and, by the next spring, she was pretty much back to normal—active and fully functioning. Most importantly, when she experiences pain related to arthritis, she knows what to do to bring relief, and when she is feeling depressed, she knows how to lift her mood. Iyengar yoga gives Jenna a feeling of joy, accomplishment, and confidence.

"Below is a portion of a letter I received from a 14-year-old yoga student:

> *Very early on, I discovered that yoga makes you fix problems yourself. It also worked much faster than any of the other treatments, and the results lasted much longer. I learned that my headaches were a result of deeper problems, and headaches were the way my body let me know something was wrong. Yoga made me fix my headaches myself, and not rely on medication or a machine to solve my problem. And if I ever get headaches again, I know what to do.*

"Iyengar yoga is a profound meditation on the body where kids—rather than avoid their problems and pain—look at the underlying causes and habits that may contribute to these problems and learn how to change them. For example, if a child has chronic headaches, it is quite possible that her neck and shoulders will be tight and contracted into a hard knot. She may have a rounded upper back and throw her head forward. She will probably be completely unaware of how much tension she is holding in her neck and how it is affected by her posture.

"Yoga is not just a series of exercises simply designed to build strength and flexibility. It is a vehicle for developing awareness. It is a process that develops strength of will, trust, confidence, and a willingness to look at one's self without judgment. Kids who practice Iyengar yoga for their chronic pain problems begin to see that they have some control over the underlying causes of their problems. Even kids who have conditions like rheumatoid arthritis, which yoga cannot cure, learn to see that yoga practice can greatly decrease or eliminate pain and reduce flareups. By doing yoga, those who feel betrayed by their bodies can learn some mastery over their problems and, by their own actions, develop a sense of competence and control.

"The young people who come to our pediatric pain program—and likely those who visit other similar pain programs—have typically sought medical help repeatedly without benefit. They are particularly vulnerable to feeling depressed and hopeless. We have observed the positive effect that Iyengar yoga has on their mood."

We have begun to carry out research on the effects of yoga in young people. In our first study, we learned that Iyengar yoga not only can improve mood and function but is also associated with a reduction in the body's major stress hormone (Woolery A, Myers H, Sternlieb B, Zeltzer LK: A yoga intervention for young adults with elevated symptoms of depression, *Alternative Therapies in Health & Medicine*, 2004; 10:60–63).

It is best to learn Iyengar yoga with a qualified teacher. To find a teacher near you, consult the Web site of the Iyengar Yoga National Association of the United States at www.iynaus.org/. You can also call your local yoga studios and ask if they have a certified Iyengar yoga teacher on staff. When you speak to the teacher, make sure you share with her your child's relevant medical history so that she can assess the most effective and safe way for your child to begin a yoga practice.

HYPNOTHERAPY

In the mid-1970s, as a fellow in adolescent medicine at Childrens Hospital Los Angeles, I was curious about why some adolescents with chronic disease had a lot of symptoms, such as pain, whereas others with the same disease had few symptoms. This curiosity led to my exploration into how the mind and body worked together to create or reduce symptoms. It was amazing to me how thoughts, images, or emotions could actually affect pain, nausea, vomiting, and other physical symptoms. I started reading about different ways that the mind might influence the body and came across some books and articles on hypnosis.

I joined the Society for Clinical and Experimental Hypnosis (SCEH) to learn more, and because I wanted to start using hypnotherapy with my patients, I asked a local SCEH member who had a lot of clinical experience if he would supervise me in my hypnotherapy work. This clinical supervisor, Dr. Martin Reiser, was at the time the chief psychologist at the Los Angeles Police Department, and he had been using hypnotherapy with police officers to help them with headaches, stress, and other symptoms.

Soon after, I attended a workshop on hypnosis and pain at the annual meeting of the SCEH. Dr. Paul Sacerdote, a psychologist who was the workshop leader, had asked for patient volunteers with whom to demonstrate techniques of hypnosis. I invited an older teenage patient of mine, Gerald, to come to the meeting.

* * *

Gerald had SCD with recurrent bouts of pain. (He was called a "frequent flyer" by the other pediatric residents because of his frequent use of the ER for Demerol shots for pain episodes.)

Dr. Sacerdote had Gerald in a deep hypnotic state in a matter of minutes. He urged Gerald to relax and breathe deeply, taking in more oxygen. He told Gerald that his mind would "know" when a sickle cell crisis was about to come and that his mind would help him take deep breaths at those times to prevent the sickle cell crisis. (Low oxygen can precipitate a sickle cell crisis and giving oxygen can help during a sickle cell crisis, but there are no studies documenting the prevention of a crisis by breathing deeply). Gerald left the meeting feeling "different," but he couldn't explain how or why.

Gerald had previously been meeting with me for hypnotherapy sessions in which he would go to his "favorite place" (usually that meant with his girlfriend anywhere). He had always felt relaxed at the sessions, but nothing special had happened to his sickle cell pain episodes. However, during our next session after his experience with Dr. Sacerdote, rather than going to a "favorite place" that consisted of imagining being with his girl-friend, Gerald began to have images of sewers overrun by rats, and a huge hose with high-pressure water that would wash out the rats and garbage.

In his hypnotherapy sessions with me, he continued to imagine this set of images. He explained that these images came to him when I asked him to imagine what happened in his body during a sickle cell pain episode and to imagine what he would need to do in order to "undo" the pain episode. After four months, Gerald was going to the ER less often and was taking lower doses of pain medication.

* * *

Several years later, Gerald received training as an emergency medical technician and became the first ambulance driver with SCD in Los Angeles.

I asked J. Kathryn de Planque, Ph.D., the hypnotherapist in our pain program, to describe what she says to parents when a child with chronic pain first comes to see her:

"My treatment is based upon a mind–body approach to healing. Children with chronic pain generally require a calming of the nervous system. The use of hypnotherapy and guided imagery influences this process as well as provides support for strengthening the immune system, release of stress and pain, and other healing goals set by the child. Many of these goals are emotionally based, such as reducing sadness or worry. My goal is for the child to learn how to help him- or herself to heal and stay well.

"I always begin with an explanation of how the mind influences the body, and I think it is vitally important that each child, no matter what age, has a clear understanding of *why* hypnotherapy works and *how* they can use it to help themselves.

"Establishing safety and trust, especially with teenagers, is most important. I also try to instill in the children I see a sense that they can influence change within their own body by using their mind. After two or three sessions, the child begins to make his own choices of where to go, and we may agree on the goal for the day. Before six sessions, we will make a tape that is specific to the child's needs that can be used at home.

"Eight-year-old Peter wrote me a letter about a year after seeing me. He said in his letter that he uses 'the techniques every day. Whether I am depressed, sad, or just feeling normal, your tapes help. When my headache was worse, you made me feel better. . . . ' "

PHYSICAL THERAPY

I have chosen to include PT in this CAM chapter even though it is really part of the world of conventional medical treatments, because the way that we use PT is similar to the way we use other treatments discussed here. PT is especially useful—although not exclusively—for chronic musculoskeletal (myofascial) pain, CRPS, and muscular deterioration due to inactivity.

The primary role of the physical therapist is to help your child's physical structural body become normalized and in balance, including posture, tight or weak muscles, and muscle-nerve mechanics. Many physical therapists also use electrical stimulation units for treating pain. The most commonly used home device is the transcutaneous electrical nerve stimulation (TENS) unit. This is a gadget that your child can wear. It has electrodes that she can place on the part of the body that is in the most pain. The physical therapist can teach your child how to increase the frequency or amount of stimulation so that she can feel a comfortable "buzz" that doesn't hurt but feels good. This stimulation is believed to block pain signals and can be very effective for some children. It also is typically covered by most health insurances. Another device that is used in the office and can be used at home is sympathetic stimulation. This helps treat chronic pain by stimulating the CNS in a way that ultimately calms the nerves that are overactive. You can find out more about this therapy and contact a clinic near your home by going to www.chronicpainrx.com/chronicpain/dynatron.

I asked Sean Hampton, MPT, a longtime physical therapist in our UCLA pediatric pain program (and director of ADI Rehab), to talk about PT in children with chronic pain:

"While electrical stimulation can be helpful in treating chronic pain, physical therapists employ many other treatments to help your child get back to an active life. The therapist may also use manual hands-on stretching and mobilization treatments to help stretch out muscles, joints, and nerves that have become tight over time and with decreased activity. The therapist must have the ability to make therapy fun and interesting for children.

"The pediatric pain physical therapist must establish a trusting relationship with the child for many reasons. The child with chronic pain may have seen numerous professionals who may have let him down. Every chronic pain patient is told 'I will help you get rid of your pain.' When the child puts trust and hope in those promises, he may ultimately be let down when the pain does not go away. When this happens over and over, often with painful evaluations and procedures occurring along the way, the child with chronic pain may start to look at all practitioners with skepticism.

"Michelle came to see me for severe CRPS of her lower extremities and was very skeptical of all therapists, especially when it came to touching or moving her legs. She had resisted any movement of her legs with every therapist and was continuing this behavior with me. I had asked her to bend her knees and Michelle demonstrated virtually no movement with her knee. I asked Michelle if that was all she could do. Michelle said yes and wanted to know if I thought that she could bend them more than she demonstrated. Now, I had seen her move her knees more outside physical therapy. In this situation, most people and physical therapists may want to challenge a patient like this. They may choose to tell her that they saw her move her legs more before on her own. However, because Michelle had lacked trust in her previous physical therapists, she had had limited to no success with her therapy in the past. Realizing this, I knew that it was more important to gain Michelle's trust than to challenge her ability to move.

"If I had challenged her *perception* of what she was able to do or not do, Michelle would have assumed I did not believe her, that I thought she was faking her pain, and she would have grown distant and uncooperative during our sessions. I simply waited until Michelle had gained confidence in me and in her abilities. And this approach paid off; little by little, Michelle was able to do more in physical therapy, and the more she could do, the closer she came to recognizing that moving her legs was within her control. Soon she was able to acknowledge the leg movements she had been making all along. This was an exciting new discovery for Michelle."

The goal of PT is to help restore balance to the physical body and to get the child to develop a regular exercise program. Exercise strengthens muscles and improves blood circulation and body posture. It also has more general benefits; exercise can help improve range of movement, body image, movement, sleep, and mood. When a child is in pain, he may cut back on or stop exercising or participating in sports and other activities. Muscles that aren't used regularly begin to weaken and then atrophy (muscle cells die and the muscle actually gets smaller). The best way to stop this from happening is to develop an exercise program under the direction and supervision of a qualified physical therapist who understands chronic pain in children.

• • •

Karen, a fourth-grader with CRPS of her left knee, was in a wheelchair when I first saw her. She had been to other physical therapists before she came to our program, and she found PT too painful. She believed that it made her condition worse, and thus she resisted it. Karen's parents were suffering, too, from watching their daughter and were distraught, unsure whether making her go to PT was the best thing to do for their daughter. When I suggested PT as a part of the treatment plan, Karen and her parents became visibly anxious. I suggested that they just go for one visit and then they could decide if they wanted to continue. I had talked with Sean Hampton about Karen and her previous experiences with PT, and he knew that he had to form an alliance with her before she would do the necessary physical work. He spent his initial session getting to know her and finding out what her interests were. He used what he learned to develop games that interested her so that he could get her to move her body in the way that he wanted her to. He worked with Karen's family to develop motivations or rewards for when Karen reached certain milestones.

Once Karen started working with Sean, her progress was immediate. She traded her wheelchair for crutches, and soon she had no need for crutches either. Her pain significantly improved, and she was playing ball and other running games with her friends within a few months. Sean sensed that part of the original problem with PT was that Karen did not trust her own abilities and feared the pain. As he showed her that she could do certain things well without pain, PT became fun, and Karen was able to take greater and greater risks with her body. She also liked and trusted Sean, which helped her to trust herself. And by seeing her own accomplishments, she felt more capable and could do more.

• • •

Finding a qualified physical therapist is a very important yet difficult task. Unfortunately, there is currently only certification in pediatric physical therapy, but not in pediatric pain physical therapy. Try to find a physical therapist who has experience treating chronic pain, and ideally with children as well. As with all health care practitioners, the best physical therapist is one who can instill independence and confidence in a child and not base treatment on a strict protocol applied across the board to all patients. For example, Diane Poladian, one of our pain program physical therapists, used a large ball and other props to engage a young boy with belly pain and chronic fatigue who was apprehensive about PT. She turned their sessions into a game and helped him begin an exercise program that was fun. Soon he asked his parents to buy him a ball, and he began using it at home.

If you cannot find a therapist in your area with experience working with children with chronic pain, tell the therapist that you want a *gradual* reconditioning program to help your child become more active. The therapist should assess your child for muscle strength and for areas of muscle spasm and work on these areas with a series of stretching exercises.

MASSAGE

Massage is one of two therapies that account for nearly half of all visits to practitioners of CAM therapies. Massage therapy is one of the oldest methods of health care still in practice. Dr. Cynthia Myers, a massage therapist and research psychologist in our program, said that massage "involves the kneading, stroking, and manipulation of your body's soft tissues—your skin, muscles, and tendons. A massage therapist primarily uses his or her hands to manipulate muscles and tissues, but also may use his or her forearms, elbows, or feet."

Massage therapy is based on the belief that when muscles are overworked, waste products can accumulate in the muscle, causing soreness and stiffness. The therapy aims to improve circulation in the muscle, increasing flow of nutrients, and eliminating waste products. Massage can be used as part of PT, sports medicine, nursing care, or acupuncture. It may be used, for example, to relieve a child's muscle tension or promote relaxation, as the child receives other types of medical treatment. There are different forms of massage, including Swedish massage, deep tissue massage, and craniosacral therapy. The type used will depend on the child's pain problem.

Massage can reduce heart rate, relax muscles, improve range of motion in joints, and increase production of the body's natural painkillers. It also can help relieve headaches and lower blood pressure. Although massage is usually safe, it should not be done over an open wound, skin infection, phlebitis (inflammation of a vein), or in areas where bones are weak. If your child's joints are inflamed or if she has an injury, check with her doctor before she has a massage.

Nine-year-old Abe had chronic tension headaches. His mother was taught how to massage Abe's scalp, neck, shoulders, and upper back, and they developed a 15-minute massage routine before he went to sleep at night. Abe describes this experience:

• • •

> I used to get scared to go to sleep at night because I knew my head would keep hurting and I wouldn't want to be alone 'cause of the pain. Then Erin *[Erin Wilson, the pain program massage therapist]* would come to our house and rub my head and back, and that made my head stop hurting. My mom used to try to rub my head, but she rubbed too hard and it hurt. Erin taught my mom how to do it just right, and that felt sooo good that I went right to sleep.

MINDFULNESS MEDITATION

As I have been learning mindfulness meditation, a type of meditation practice, I have come to realize the value of meditation for children, parents, and families. The goal of mindfulness meditation is to help you learn how to be present and in the moment. So many of us are so worried about what we did, what happened, what we have to do, or what will happen that we spend much of our lives not enjoying or appreciating the present moment, being alive, and being with people we love. Learning mindfulness meditation helps us do this. I asked Trudy Goodman, a clinical psychologist trained in Zen and Vipassana (insight) meditation who is my meditation teacher and who works with families, to share her thoughts about meditation. When Trudy talks about mindfulness, she is referring to what happens to you in your daily life when you learn this type of meditation. (For more on specific meditation techniques, see Chapter 10, "Helping Your Child Cope with Chronic Pain.")

"I began to practice mindfulness meditation when my daughter was five years old. It was so helpful to me that I never stopped, and I have been teaching mindfulness meditation to parents and kids ever since. Mindfulness is being present with what is happening, in a balanced and nonjudgmental way. Mindfulness also helps us be with children, who are sensitive and vulnerable to acceptance or disapproval. When we parents cultivate mindful awareness, we develop more patience and acceptance when our child is in distress. This helps the whole family.

"Mindfulness helps us find the distance to be with a child in pain—if we get too close, too reactive, we are too involved—and this hurts rather than helps the child. If we seek to protect ourselves and pull too far back, our child can feel abandoned. The practice of mindfulness helps us connect with our child and stay with him. The way to do this is to return to the present moment, to the simple sensory awareness of what's going on in that moment. Our children give us feedback when we slip out of attention, if we choose to listen; they have a kind of sonar for authentic presence.

"Our mindful presence helps our children tolerate their own painful experiences with more calm. Children find out that most experiences are not as bad or as scary as they think. They rediscover how to experience directly, simply, exactly what is, even if it's unpleasant, without making a big fuss. Even when a child is going through an emotional or physical storm, a mindful parent can stay centered right in the midst of the storm. When we can reduce our own stress level and relax, our children can borrow from our strength and cope better with their own stress.

"By practicing mindfulness, we can learn to relax right in the midst of difficulties, without having to escape. We can stay empathically close to our child. Lots of times, what gets in the way of parents' being effective is the need to have things go well and the feelings of failure and frustration that come up when it doesn't happen that way. And when our children are suffering, mindfulness can make the difference between offering a wise response or an emotional reaction that we may regret. We don't have to make it all better or make it go away, but just be willing to be there, accepting, caring, and kind.

"Mindfulness meditation can decrease stress, increase our pleasure in parenting, and increase our capacity to live in the moment and to turn off the critical tapes that run in every parent's mind. Learning to relax and breathe into the moment brings a sense of confidence; kids can also learn mindfulness meditation. Sometimes the best way is for the family to learn together and practice together."

ART THERAPY

I asked Esther Dreifuss-Kattan, Ph.D., a psychoanalyst and an art therapist in our pain program, to discuss what art therapy is and how it is used for children with chronic pain:

"One of the primary goals of art therapy is to understand the internal world of children. We strive to make it accessible for exploration and then search for the meanings that will ameliorate physical and psychic pain and foster growth. If we are to communicate effectively with our patients, it is essential to discover a common language. Long before the development of language, the infant has his own world with self-created images and sensory experiences. Sigmund Freud suggested that children at play behave like creative writers or artists, developing a world that pleases them. He indicated art's curious ability to handle feelings and themes that in ordinary life are too painful to talk about directly.

"The picture is a bridge between the inner and the outer world of the child. Both worlds contribute to the creation of the picture. Through their pictures, children express and project their inner images. Once the picture is finished, the art therapist will look at the finished product with the child and invite the child artist to share his feelings, thoughts, and associations about it. However, if the patient is too young or is not interested in talking about the picture, that is fine, too. Often the act of creation is therapeutic in itself. However, if a discussion is established, the child may share with the therapist a possible title or story or explain the individual parts of the picture. The better the therapist knows the child and his or her medical, psychological, and family history, the easier it is for her to interpret some of the content of the picture. This can relieve fears, allow for exploration of trauma, and elucidate family dynamics. Art therapy allows for externalizing on the paper the internal world and conflicts of the child.

"Joe, who was referred to me through the pain clinic, was a withdrawn, stressed, 16-year-old gifted high school student with severe chronic headaches. He completed a scribble drawing in the first consultation. Filling in the colors, he recognized a bird with a huge head, with a red area, a small body, and tiny wings. Joe's chronic, severe headaches, which had made him dependent on medication, were surfacing unconsciously in the big head of this bird. Together, we realized how the oversized head made it impossible for the bird to take off and fly to his own place, away from his protective mother and the parents' marital conflicts. Joe's love of art and his ability to express his pain through his artwork and also to understand his pictures brought him joy and relief."

LAUGHTER AND HUMOR THERAPY

I became interested in the science of laughter and humor, and especially its potential role in the treatment of children with chronic pain, after I met Sherry Dunay Hilber, who was a prime-time TV program executive involved with top situation comedies. She noticed that laughing seemed to induce a domino effect of good moods in the people with whom she worked. This interest in the benefits of humor and comedy viewing led her to explore the roles of humor and laughter in the health and well-being of children. She said, "I wanted to know if there was a practical application for comedy viewing, such as in the form of a physician's 'prescription' for sick children to watch a certain amount of comedy to aid in their recovery." Sherry met with UCLA child psychiatrist Dr. Margaret Stuber and me to develop research on laughter and children's pain. We developed a pilot study that found that watching a funny video reduced children's laboratory pain responses and lowered their levels of the stress hormone cortisol. We are continuing this research. (For more information, go to www.rxlaughter.org.)

ENERGY THERAPY

Energy therapy, bioenergy, therapeutic touch, Reiki, and healing touch are the five CAM categories described by NCCAM to refer to a system of nontouch (or light touch) healing treatments. Energy therapies assume the existence of a field of energy originating from within the body. Energy therapists perceive blocks or depletions within the patient's body. These blocks are assumed to be energetic reflections of pain.

The therapist manipulates the energy field with his or her hands to enhance the flow of energy, restoring and clearing these disturbances. Most energy practices have the underlying belief that illness occurs on the vibrational level before solidifying and manifesting in the body. It is believed that this life force is inherent to health and flows freely and fully when health is present. Energy therapists believe that as illness begins to settle into the body, the flow of this life substance begins to slow, stagnate, and become blocked. Energy therapy attempts to break up these blocks or unhealthy patterns both before and after illness is present and allow health to return to the body, mind, and emotions of the patient.

Some therapists work with the various systems of the body identified by Western medicine, such as the nervous, endocrine, and lymphatic systems, as well as the major organs of the body. Others work with bodily systems identified by Eastern medicine, including the chakras and the meridians (see the section entitled "Acupuncture" earlier in this chapter), which also correspond to the various organs and systems in allopathic (mainstream Western) medicine.

Dr. Audrey Easton, who was our energy clinician before she moved to India, describes her work this way:

"Sessions begin with a brief discussion with the child or her parents. I ask what the child's current symptoms are and how much pain or discomfort she has. I explain what energy healing is and discover whether the child has any concerns. Generally, the child lies on a table on his or her back fully clothed, but without shoes. I stand or sit in a chair behind the child's head and assume a meditative, calm, peaceful state. I bring my hands within a few inches of the child's head and attempt to connect with the child's energy field. Energy healing is very different from massage or other types of body work in that there is very little actual manipulation or even contact with the child's body. I hold my hands still, over the child's body, until I feel a shift (calming) in the child's energy. If there is a serious blockage in the child's energy body, one of my hands may serve as a conduit for the energy while the other may act as a receptor of the energetic blocks in the child. I may move my hands over the child's head and upper body, exploring energy blocks and allowing a flow to occur. I may stand up and move either to the child's feet or torso. If a particular organ or physiological system is known to be impaired, I may work directly at that source. The session ends with my returning to the head, establishing a consistent flow of energy throughout the entire system. I touch the child's shoulders, indicating the treatment is over.

"A nine-year-old girl with fibromyalgia, formerly a gymnast, was in such pain when she came to see me that she could no longer do any exercise. I can remember her vivid description of the treatment. When I was working over her knees, she said, 'It feels like my knees are in a microwave!' Later, at her throat: 'It feels like there are fireflies in my throat.' At the end of the session, she jumped up and screamed, 'Mommy, Daddy, I feel better!' "

{ CHAPTER NINE }

Individual and Family Therapy

There is no coming to consciousness without pain.
—CARL JUNG

Tom is a bright and witty 12-year-old with recurring abdominal pain. His pains reliably occurred every weekday morning when he had to get ready for school. Tom's morning pain symptoms often involved crying and screaming. His pains had caused him to miss significant amounts of school, but they usually improved by the late afternoon, at which time he would go to play outside with his friends. Tom had developed anxieties about going to school, partly as a result of his mother's belief that the school staff was not sympathetic to his pain problems. Tom was convinced that he could not be at school and cope with his pain at the same time.

The first goal of family therapy was to change Tom's mother's perceptions about the school by developing an agreement (a signed contract) among the school principal, nurse, Tom, and his mother, stating that Tom would be allowed certain privileges at school (e.g., lying down in the nurse's office when he was in pain). In return, Tom's mother was to get Tom to school every day. In the beginning, the plan was for Tom to remain at school through first period. His time at school was increased gradually each week and he received incentives for his ability to cope with being in school, such as going outside to play with his friends.

Soon Tom's mother was able to get him to school and was less anxious about what might happen to him while he was there. In turn, once Tom sensed his mother's changing attitude toward the school and became confident in his own ability to stay at school for increasing amounts of time, he was able to go to school more easily, he became interested in some of his classes, and his pain lessened.

INDIVIDUAL AND GROUP THERAPY

When a child has a pain problem that is not responding to medications, many physicians will say that the child should see a mental health specialist, suggesting that the problem is not a physical one but a mental one. But as I've explained in defining pain–brain interaction, pain is neither purely physical nor purely psychological. So when is psychotherapy helpful? This chapter answers this and other questions you may have regarding individual and family therapy.

In Chapter 5, "Factors That Contribute to Chronic Pain," I discussed certain factors that can cause a pain problem to worsen if they are not addressed. In this chapter, we revisit some of those factors (such as anxiety, depression, coping problems, social skills deficits, and others) and see how to address them with individual and/or family therapy. Some pain problems can be helped with only medication, but often psychotherapy alone or with medication and various complementary therapies works best. Also, unlike when a child's pain is being treated with medication alone, psychotherapy helps your child to build skills so that he can help himself.

Sometimes children have problems coping with day-to-day events. They may view certain situations as overwhelming or just avoid activities that they feel they cannot handle. These children give up readily in dealing with daily hassles, so when larger problems come up, they just retreat and leave the problem to someone else, typically a parent, to solve. This passive coping style is especially problematic when these children have to tackle a pain problem. Psychotherapy may be aimed at helping children with poor coping abilities to develop more positive ways of appraising or viewing situations and to handle them in a more satisfying way.

● ● ●

Glenn is a 14-year-old who suffered with headaches. The headaches were causing him to sleep so poorly that he said that he was always tired during the day. Sometimes he was so tired that he refused to go to school because he just "couldn't get out of bed." At other times, he said that his headaches were too bad to allow him to go to school.

Glenn began missing more and more school. When he did go to school, he had two "sort of" friends, the computer geek and the math whiz. However, he found school stressful because he had difficulty relating to most of the other kids, whom he thought were all "too dumb."

An evaluation of Glenn indicated symptoms of Asperger's. He was very smart, excelling in math and computer science, and there were other signs for this diagnosis. He was very logical and could be very argumentative, often not giving up in an argument at home until he drove his parents crazy. We realized that the stressful part of school for Glenn was the social in-

teraction rather than the academic work. He was referred for social skills training in a group format so that he would learn some
of the social skills that didn't come naturally to him. For example, he had to learn how to let others children "be right" some of
the time and not argue them to death. He had to learn how to
make eye contact and smile more, especially if other children
smiled at him. He got to practice these skills with other kids similar to him, and they all learned together.

An incremental plan was established for Glenn to go back
to school full-time, and he learned biofeedback to control the
muscle tension that contributed to his headaches. With the combination of biofeedback, social skills training, and a school reen-
try plan, Glenn was able to fall asleep better on school nights,
awaken more easily in the mornings, and eventually attend
school full-time. In the group therapy, he also learned how to
participate in school in ways that took advantage of what he was
good at—he joined the debate team and set up "mind-game puz-
zles" on the computer for the school newspaper. (Typically only
he and his two other friends could figure out the answers, and he
loved that!)

ANXIETY DISORDERS AND
COGNITIVE-BEHAVIORAL THERAPY

I often refer children with anxiety problems to a cognitive-behavioral
therapist. In CBT, children learn: to identify situations that make them
anxious, to change the way they think about situations (this is called cognitive reframing), and to reduce their feelings of anxiety at those times,
through various relaxation and mental strategies. Behavior therapy helps
children to identify and address different situations that cause them stress
and pain and helps them to adopt new ways to react. It also teaches them
how to be calm so that they can feel better, think more clearly, and make
better decisions.

• • •

Angela is a 13-year-old with IBS that was causing her such severe belly pain that she was unable to return to school after the winter holiday. She also had GAD (lots of chronic worrying about missing school, falling behind, not getting A's, not being able to make the basketball team, her parents' health, her father's job, her sister's asthma, etc.). Angela began focusing on her belly pain in the mornings before school. According to her, she "tried to go to school" but was unable to, and she worried that even if she forced herself to go, she would never be able to stay in school because of her pain. Soon she began worrying the night before school. All of these worries made her pain worse and worse. She was missing more and more school and getting further behind. Because Angela had been a straight-A student and was a perfectionist, she worried constantly about falling behind and not being able to get A's. We referred Angela to a psychologist for CBT.

The psychologist first helped Angela figure out what kinds of situations made her feel tense and have more pain. Angela realized that it wasn't school in general that made her anxious, but some bullies at school who had made fun of her just before the winter break. She had not been back to school since. She had identified a significant and specific problem that was stressful for her.

Angela learned some strategies to reduce her anxiety when she thought about going to school and seeing these students. She learned a technique known as thought-stopping. When she began thinking catastrophic thoughts (e.g., *They are going to laugh at me and get everyone in the school to laugh at me*), she would tell herself, *Stop. . . . This is not going to happen. . . . I can handle seeing them.*

Angela also learned some breathing exercises to calm herself when she felt her heart beginning to race or her hands becoming sweaty. She developed a plan for what she would do at school when she saw the other students and figured out how she might react in a couple of different scenarios, depending on how the girls behaved toward her (e.g., if they looked at her, laughed, pushed her, etc.).

Angela practiced this plan in her mind first and then role-played it with her therapist. She was able to go to school, and even though the girls laughed at her, as she had feared, she was prepared for it, and she was able to ignore them and feel okay. This made it easier for her to return to school the next day. As her stress about going to school lessened and she felt more competent, her belly pain also got better and she was able to easily get caught up in the work she had missed and continued to make all A's.

· · ·

Often in CBT, children first practice being able to think about the things that make them anxious and then think or imagine themselves in the situation. Then little by little, they practice actually doing the thing(s) that makes them anxious. This practice of accomplishing a task in small increments is called *desensitization*. Relaxation training, hypnotherapy, and mindfulness meditation (see Chapter 8, "Complementary and Alternative Therapies") can also be incorporated into CBT to help a child desensitize herself so that she can function well, worry less, and feel better overall.

DEPRESSION AND COPING

Chronic pain can lead to depression, and depression can reduce a child's ability to cope with pain. Although medications such as antidepressants can be helpful in children with depression, these children often need the kind of help that you can't find in a bottle of pills. One teen with chronic muscle pain reported feeling so sad at night that she would cry secretly in her bedroom—too distraught and embarrassed to ask her parents for help, she was trying to handle it on her own. She also thought that if she told her parents how hopeless she felt her pain situation had become and how helpless she felt, they would think she was weak. She had always prided herself on being the strong one in the family. It wasn't until she started to have thoughts about killing herself that she became frightened enough to tell her parents. They were understanding and brought her to a psychotherapist.

Almost all children in pain at one time or another wish they weren't alive. However, if you take time to listen to them, what they typically mean is that they wish that they didn't have to live with their pain. This is different from thinking about killing themselves, which is called suicidal ideation (thinking). If your child appears depressed, it is important to talk with her and find out some details—for example: Has she thought about dying? About killing herself? About how she would kill herself? Has she made preparations for her suicide (notes, giving possessions away, gathering pill bottles, etc.)? If your child attempts suicide or tells you about details of planning for a suicide, then you need to bring your child to an ER for psychiatric evaluation to see how imminent the danger is. The psychiatric evaluation will determine whether hospitalization is needed for your child's protection or whether your child is safe to return home and begin psychotherapy.

SOCIAL SKILLS TRAINING

Some children need to learn how to interact with other kids. They may have a difficult time at school because of the social setting rather than the academics. They may be shy or they may just not know what to do in social situations. For example, imagine that two children on the playground at school see a group of kids from their class talking together. One child might worry that the other kids are talking about him and want to avoid the group, and then come home feeling rejected. The other child might see the same group of kids and approach them, smiling, and ask them what they are doing and if he can join in. It is the same situation experienced in two very different ways.

As I discussed in Chapter 6 ("Pervasive Developmental Disorders"), some children, such as those with PDDs, have a difficult time reading the facial expressions or other nonverbal behavior of others. The part of their brain that interprets the meaning of behavior and understands social etiquette is not working well. This is the child who is avoided at school because he comes up to other kids and stands almost on top of them. He is not aware of personal space or that he is making others uncomfortable by standing too close. This is the child who may say hurtful things to other kids without even realizing it.

These children need to be taught social interaction skills that don't come naturally, such as when you stand by another person, make sure that you stand at least an arm's distance away. Or, when you talk with someone, it is important to look the person in the eyes. Children who have a difficult time understanding the intentions of others can be taught how to ask if they don't understand what has been said. Social skills training is best taught in a peer group setting so that children can get direct feedback from other children about their behaviors and responses.

IDENTIFYING COMMUNICATION PROBLEMS

Children with a disorder called alexithymia have problems identifying and labeling their emotions. They might have difficulty knowing whether they are feeling sad, anxious, or angry. For these children, negative emotions that remain unidentified, unexpressed, and therefore untreated can aggravate a pain problem. In this case, therapy teaches children what emotions feel like. The ability to understand your own emotional state is important in both seeking support and in engaging with others in general. Another kind of communication problem that benefits from therapy is verbal expression problems. Some children know what they mean and want to say but have difficulty expressing themselves and finding the right words to say what they mean. This difficulty can create great stress for a child and can magnify an existing pain problem.

ADDRESSING UNRESOLVED GRIEF OR TRAUMA

Children who have suffered a loss, such as a family member, friend, or even a pet, will go through a normal mourning period. However, with some children, this grief continues beyond what might be considered normal and interferes with functioning or leads to profound feelings of sadness. In this case, psychotherapy can be very useful in helping the child to weather the mourning process and feel better.

Children who have experienced or witnessed a trauma (earthquake, shooting, physical or sexual abuse) can suffer from PTSD and can have sleep disturbances, flashbacks of the event, and intrusive thoughts; can be emotionally numb; and may startle easily. PTSD will invariably make pain worse and harder to treat and will interfere with a child's life in many ways. Children with PTSD should ideally see a therapist trained in modern methods of treating PTSD, because many advances have been made in our understanding and treatment of this condition in recent years.

• • •

Faith is a 10-year-old who had had a successful heart transplant. However, she had many postoperative problems, especially with one of the catheters that carried blood in and out of her body. It had to be replaced once and she had a lot of painful surgical manipulation in that area of her body. When she was last in the hospital, before I first saw her, the catheter fell out while she was in the bathroom alone and she started bleeding and became panicked. Her anxiety rose quickly, and the pain circuits relating to her catheter site became turned on; she immediately developed severe lower belly pain near the area where her catheter had been. The catheter was replaced, but the pain continued. None of the cardiologists or surgeons could figure out what was causing the pain, even after many tests. Because they couldn't find a fixable cause, they didn't know what to do to reduce her pain. When they gave her typical opioid pain medicines, she would just go to sleep, awakening still in pain. Fortunately for Faith, these doctors understood their own limitations in pain treatment and referred her to our program.

We diagnosed Faith's condition as PTSD resulting from her many surgical procedures and especially from the bleeding episode in the bathroom. The PTSD had caused a change in her neural arousal system so that even low levels of pain were hard for her to bear, and she had flashbacks of the bleeding episode, trouble sleeping, and intrusive thoughts about her hospital experiences. The pain signals from her catheter site kept sending pain signals to her brain in a neural loop that kept the pain going.

We used one medication to calm her heightened nervous system and PTSD symptoms and another aimed at her nerve hyperexcitability. We then referred Faith to a psychologist who would help her to talk about her stressful hospital experience and to face her fears. She learned skills to overcome the anxiety she felt when she thought about that experience, and over time, she was able to revisit the hospital ward and feel okay there. Currently, Faith is taking very little pain and anxiety-related medications. She is going to school, has friends, and is physically active. She no longer constantly worries about her heart or being hospitalized.

FAMILY THERAPY AND BEHAVIORAL PLANS

Marvin is a three-year-old boy who was scheduled to have his second heart surgery. His first surgery a year earlier was difficult and caused distress for Marvin and anxiety for his parents. His postoperative pain was not managed well, and as a result, he became extremely anxious about going back into the hospital. His parents were very worried that Marvin would be in a lot of pain after this surgery. I asked my psychology graduate student, Lauren, to meet Marvin and his parents and see how she might be able to help.

Lauren met the family, and they developed a plan together. First, she engaged Marvin in play therapy for a few days prior to the surgery. Marvin pretended to be the doctor and used a "poker" to give Lauren several shots. Marvin acted out his fears about the surgery, and Lauren provided him with more realistic information about the surgery in age-appropriate ways (e.g., "You are going to come with your mommy and daddy, and you get to bring your favorite stuffed animal. Whom are you going to bring? Teddy? Great! He will feel so soft and cuddly. Then you and Teddy and your mommy and daddy will meet the doctor. He will be wearing a funny green suit with a really funny hat. The hat might even make you laugh, it is so funny.").

Lauren also worked with Marvin's parents to develop a tape of Marvin's mother reading his favorite stories and singing songs. The tape was played as Marvin was being taken into the operating room (with his mother and Teddy also present until he was sedated), during the surgery, and in the postoperative aftercare unit.

Marvin's parents reported that he appeared much calmer as he went into surgery than he had the previous time. His mother reminded him about the doctor's (anesthesiologist's) funny green hat, and they all laughed together, including the anesthesiologist.

Lauren also spent time talking with Marvin's parents about their own anxieties. Children often are sensitive to parental anxiety and use their parents' reactions as a cue for how they should be reacting. In addition, certain adult behaviors such as apologies, reassurance, and criticism, are typically associated with increased child distress. Because of her mistrust of the doctors' ability to manage

Marvin's pain, Marvin's mother was frequently apologetic when Marvin complained of pain and would reassure him that "everything will be okay." She was encouraged instead to help distract Marvin by engaging him in play or telling him stories.

Marvin recovered quickly from his surgery and displayed much less anxiety after this surgery than after the previous one. He required minimal postoperative pain medication and had a much shorter hospital stay than the previous time.

• • •

Marvin's story illustrates how a behavioral plan can be developed and implemented and, in this case, how such a plan made the surgical experience for Marvin better and reduced his parents' anxiety. For many children with chronic pain, a simple behavioral plan that addresses specific problems and sets a few goals for parents and child, such as helping the child return to school or increase his functioning in other ways, may be all that is needed. For more pervasive problems, family therapy may be needed to help the family understand that how they interact may be maintaining the child's pain or making it worse. Changing the ways that family members communicate with one another and understanding roles that individual members of a family play that maintain maladaptive family systems can be a pivotal part of the treatment program for some children with chronic pain. What goes on in the family unit can and does influence how a child responds to pain, how long it lasts, how the child copes, and, ultimately, how quickly he gets better. Families (this includes parents, siblings, and even grandparents) who understand, or are taught to understand, the important role of the family in helping a child with chronic pain to function and conquer the pain will thrive.

A child with chronic pain can also add stress to the entire family. Family outings may have to be canceled, and siblings may resent the extra attention given to the child in pain. Chronic pain is one of the top reasons why children miss school.

"Life cannot be put on hold until chronic pain goes away," says

Gary Walco, Ph.D., director of the David Center for Children's Pain and Palliative Care at Hackensack University Medical Center. "School is where children learn to get along with others and learn to problem-solve. There is no substitution for that setting, and therefore school attendance is imperative."

When your child stays home from school, you or your spouse or partner may have to miss work or scramble for child-care arrangements. Parents often have different ways of dealing with a child who reports too much pain to be able to attend school. Marital stresses can develop, siblings can behave disruptively, and the family can become stressed. Through family (or sometime just couples) therapy, families can work together to help themselves function better as a cohesive and supportive unit and, in turn, help the child with pain to function and feel better.

The goals of family therapy are to:

- Observe, identify, and alter family dynamics that may contribute to the child's pain perception and difficulty coping
- Participate in developing and implementing a behavioral plan
- Address family stress and other problems
- Improve family communication
- Provide support and improve family coping

There is often resistance to family therapy. It is easier to focus on the child with the pain problem than to examine factors that may be contributing to the problem. Parents often do not realize the inadvertent roles that they play in helping their child cross the line from having a moderate pain problem to having a pain-associated disability syndrome, a condition in which children with chronic pain quickly spiral out of control and become low-functioning or nonfunctioning.

Fortunately, parents can also help their child to become fully functional again. "Parents are an essential part of the treatment team with unique insights into their child's strengths, weaknesses, and coping style, and their enthusiastic support is at least as important as any other intervention in helping children with chronic and persistent pain problems," says Dr. Neil Schechter, director of the Pain Relief Program at Connecticut Children's Medical Center.

In the years that I have been working with children with chronic pain and their parents, I have come up with an informal list of unhelpful behaviors that parents engage in that seem to influence the degree to which their children with chronic pain are disabled by the pain. I tell you this not to make you feel like a bad parent—because you are not—but to illustrate how a parent can unknowingly add to a child's suffering so that you can do something about it by changing your behavior. These unhelpful behaviors include:

- Providing an undue amount of sympathy and attention for your child's pain complaints
- Being excessively emotional in response to your child's pain complaints and behaviors
- Continually looking for help outside the family to make your child's pain better (e.g., bringing your child to doctor after doctor for more and more tests)
- Complaining a lot about your own pain or problems, and generally showing yourself to be a poor coping example for your child
- Not functioning when you are in pain
- Supporting your child's tendency to avoid everyday tasks and responsibilities (e.g., doing chores and schoolwork) because of the pain

When should you consider family therapy? Any family can benefit from family counseling, which, in addition to redirecting behavior, will educate you about how pain works and what you can do to help your child become fully functioning again. However, I typically recommend family therapy when it appears that individual therapy is not helping or when there is clearly a family dynamic that is inhibiting the child from getting better. The general rule of thumb is that if things don't improve with adequate treatment of your child's pain, you should be considering what family factors might be inadvertently contributing to the pain. For example, take a look at yourself and your spouse or partner and notice how you or both of you react to your child when she is complaining about pain:

- Do you find that you get so anxious that you feel the need to do something immediately to make it stop?
- Do you feel that you are suffering as much as your child? Is your suffering interfering with your life and causing you to lose sleep, or have you become irritable, depressed, or anxious?
- Do you find it difficult to convince your child to do anything when he is in pain?
- Do you have a hard time *not* asking your child how she is feeling?
- Do you constantly monitor your child's face for *signs* of pain?
- Are you and your spouse or partner constantly in conflict over the best way to deal with your child?
- Are you sleeping with your child every night because he is complaining about pain?
- Do you identify too closely with your child because you have the same type of pain problem, and is it interfering with your child's ability to do things for himself?
- Do you feel that you are the one shouldering all the responsibility for your child's pain and that you are not getting the support you need from your spouse or partner?
- Are your other children starting to show signs of neglect? Are they acting out?

If your answer is yes to several of these questions, then you and your family are probably candidates for family therapy. Family therapy, which should include the entire family, is focused on changing the family system within which the child with pain is trying to cope. The therapist observes each member's perceptions of the child in pain, as well as the roles and behaviors of each family member within the family structure. In this process, the therapist will learn what factors are contributing to the child's pain experience and behaviors. For example, in some families, the child in pain is inadvertently forced to maintain the role of the "nonfunctioning pain kid" so that the focus of parental attention is off more serious and pressing family problems.

I have found that in some cases, family therapy is more important than other therapies aimed at the pain treatment itself. Stepping back from the situation and taking a good, hard, honest look at yourself and your family is not easy. In fact, of all the recommendations that I make to help a child with chronic pain get better—and they aren't all so easy—I think that my recommendation for family therapy may be the most difficult for many families to accept.

When I suggest family therapy as part of a child's treatment plan, many parents feel that I am saying that they are failures as parents. They may say, "I think we are doing pretty well. . . . Why would we need family therapy?" A recommendation for family therapy does not necessarily mean that your marriage is bad or your family is dysfunctional. Typically, the recommendation simply means that there are some behavioral patterns within the family that may be making it more difficult for the child with pain to function. Nobody is at fault; the system just needs tweaking. I can promise you that whenever a family makes the commitment to therapy, changes happen.

Eighteen-year-old Jennie reflects on when she was 10 years old, had CRPS, and was in a wheelchair because her legs hurt too much to walk:

•   •   •

I have an older brother and an older sister. It was very difficult. My brother was a freshman and my sister was going off to university. It was an important time in their lives, and a lot of my parents' attention was focused on me, and I was completely dependent on them for my movement. . . . I couldn't do anything on my own. . . . I couldn't go to the bathroom on my own. I think there was some resentment, definitely, but they never showed it. But I am sure it was difficult for them to accept.

We went to family therapy. It was difficult. But the sessions were helpful. It made my parents more aware that my brother and sister needed extra attention. It was an opportunity for me to tell them what I was going through, at a time when it wasn't an argument or a fight. It was okay for them to say, "I am angry that this is happening."

I think one of the reasons I have recovered is because of my parents. My parents gave me my space and independence as much as they could. We had just moved to California from Canada two years earlier, and all our family was in Canada, so they didn't have a support system to get a break from things. They were extremely patient. They never blamed me; they understood I was in pain.

As much as it was a difficult time in my life, if I could, I wouldn't change a thing. I consider that I am the person I am today because of what I went through. I have an incredible relationship with my parents, especially my mom, because we spent so much time together. We went through so much emotionally and physically together that it's just a really special relationship.

I am studying psychology and am debating whether I want to go to medical school. It's kind of funny, because at the time I hated the psychologist—she was the tough one. Getting me to talk was torture. I was the kid who was the pleaser. I didn't want to cause any problems. I didn't want to talk about the things that were bothering me—my depression or my anger. Those are the things I needed to do. I kept a diary as a release. I didn't keep track of improvements, because then I felt bad, like I wasn't trying hard enough, if I regressed a bit. But having a place to release emotionally was helpful. At one point I was keeping track of how many steps I could do on the crutches, and I really didn't like that. If I had a bad day, it ended up stressing me out more if I was keeping track.

• • •

It takes a lot of courage to allow a stranger to join your family circle and hear the kinds of conversations that have only taken place behind closed doors. Most importantly, it can feel threatening to allow another adult to have influence in your child's life. What if the therapist does not understand your point of view? What if the therapist contradicts you in front of your children or your spouse?

The therapist typically tries to discover what each member of the family sees as the problems and the goals that each member wants to address in family therapy. Usually some rules of therapy are discussed, such as these: Only one person talks at a time, no hitting or other physically aggressive behavior is permitted, and the whole family must be willing to attend. You should be able to share your concerns at the first session and ask as many questions as you need to in order to feel more comfortable. When you start therapy, it is important to identify what you want to get out of the experience. Your initial goal may be as broad as "I want to help my child feel better."

In preparation for writing this book, I asked many of my patients and their parents to tell me how psychotherapy helped them. Here are some of their comments:

- "I gained more confidence in my ability to tell my parents how I felt. . . . I didn't have to keep my feelings inside."

- "It was reassuring to know that if we had trouble handling something during the week, we could bring the problems up in the family session."
- "When we try to talk about some issues at home, tempers get hot. It feels safer to try [to] tackle these issues with a therapist present."
- "At least I know that there is one time a week when the family is together. With our different schedules, it seems we keep missing each other."
- "I get to hear from my daughter who doesn't have a pain problem in these meetings."
- "The therapist helps our children speak up more easily."
- "We learned to stop the blame game."

MARITAL (COUPLES) ISSUES

A family therapist may choose to work with the parents alone if she feels that this is where the primary problem is. For example, marital/couples therapy may be the most effective treatment if parental discord is creating tensions at home and aggravating the child's pain problem. The focus of marital therapy in this context is to help both parents examine their goals and expectations of their child and learn how to work together.

A couple's relationship can be strained by a child's chronic pain, so sometimes it is helpful for the parents to meet in sessions without the children. Parents may have different ways of coping with their child's pain problem, which may lead to conflicts about how to treat the child. The parents I have spoken to feel that having an opportunity to discuss these differences privately with a therapist helps them resolve their conflicts and present a more united front to the child.

When there is so much focus on children, some parents find that they neglect themselves and their partner, and their relationship suffers. They tend to become distant. It is important to set aside some specific time each week to nourish the marital relationship.

Divorced parents may find themselves having increased contact with each other as they try to help the child in pain. They may have to come together to make important decisions about their child's treatment. If divorced parents want to have an equal say in their child's health care, it is important to obtain joint legal custody in the divorce agreement. In joint legal custody, both parents have the right and the responsibility to make decisions relating to the health, education, and welfare of their child. If one parent has sole legal custody, the other parent does not have a right to make these decisions.

At UCLA, members of our legal department told me that I could not give a mother information about her child's diagnosis or treatment because the child's father had sole legal custody and refused to give us permission to talk with her. This was very difficult for the child and was a factor in their child's pain problem.

INCLUDING FATHERS

Diane Bass, L.C.S.W., our former clinic social worker, helped do some of the interviews for this book. She commented that she almost always spoke to the child's mother. She said that on a few occasions, the father would answer the phone but would quickly pass the phone to his wife, saying that she was the one to talk to. On one occasion, during her conversation with a mother, Diane heard the father calling out suggestions in the background.

Sometimes dads take a backseat when medical problems arise. They may not feel that they need to come to family therapy, especially if the mom has been the primary caregiver. This may be due to the father's own reluctance or to the mother's tendency to automatically take over, leaving the father to question what more he can do or say.

However, fathers are crucial participants in family therapy. They can provide a different point of view that balances the mother's perspective. Because fathers tend to be more objective and less protective than mothers (this is not always the case; of course, the roles can be reversed), dads can often more easily convince their child to become more independent and to cope better with the pain. The important thing is that if there are two parents (or caregivers) in the family, it is crucial to have them both take part in family therapy, especially if there are conflicts at home over what the parents expect from the child. If parents have different expectations about the way a child is handling the pain or how quickly he is recovering, the child may feel he needs to take sides, and one parent may become the "good" parent and the other "the "bad" parent. This is the kind of issue that can be worked out if both parents participate in therapy. The ultimate goal of family therapy is to establish better communication within the family.

A few words about choosing a therapist: The first place to begin is by looking at the list of mental health providers covered by your health plan. Your child's physician may know child therapists to whom he has referred children and whom he thinks are especially good. The therapist should be a licensed clinical child psychologist, child psychiatrist, licensed clinical social worker, or a licensed marriage and family therapist. You should ask about the therapist's training, credentials, and experience, especially in treating children who have chronic pain. You and your child also should like and feel connected to the psychotherapist, especially after several sessions. For guidance in finding a family therapist, see http://www.aamft.org/TherapistLocator/ (the Web site of the American Association of Marriage and Family Therapists) or http://www.apa.org/ (the Web site of the American Psychological Association).

PART IV

Parents Take Control

{ CHAPTER TEN }

Helping Your Child Cope with Chronic Pain

Good parents give their children Roots and Wings. Roots to know where home is, wings to fly away and exercise what's been taught them.

—JONAS SALK

In this chapter, we explore how to use specific techniques such as breathing and muscle relaxation, self-hypnosis, and meditation. *I can't emphasize strongly enough that it is important for you, the parent, to learn these techniques first before you teach them to your child.* Remember that you are a role model for your child. The more you look after yourself and give yourself time to relax and learn coping strategies, the more likely your child will do the same. I have written most of the explanations for you, not for your child, so you may want to adapt them a bit, depending on the age of your child. So learn well and enjoy!

You can also find strategies here for helping your child get a good night's sleep, for coping when your child has a bad pain day, and for ensuring that your child gets good medical care. Remember that the goal for the treatment of children with chronic pain is not to get rid of the pain first but rather to help them function so that the pain will then fade. Though doctors use medicines and other therapies to calm the nervous system and alter pain circuits in the brain, it's up to you to help your child carry out the tasks of daily living, including getting a good night's sleep, eating well, going to school, doing schoolwork, socializing, exercising, and participating in family activities, including home chores. Most parents want to help their child to function but don't know what to do. This chapter gives you the tools to help your child.

These relaxation techniques are ones that you and your child can use throughout life, even when there is no pain. Susmita Kashikar-Zuck, Ph.D., a psychologist in the Division of Pain Management at Cincinnati Children's Hospital Medical Center, offers this simile: "Practicing your relaxation and biofeedback skills is like a fire drill. Fires don't happen very often, but you don't want to wait until one happens to practice how to save yourself. Pain can come and go, but the time the pain is bothering you is not a good time to learn anything. You need to practice all the time so when the pain comes, you will be ready."

BREATHING EXERCISES

Depending on how it is done, breathing may reduce pain or accentuate it. Improper breathing techniques can greatly increase the pain. Some children hyperventilate when they become anxious or during a pain episode. This means that their breathing pattern changes to shallow, rapid breathing. When this happens, your child breathes out too much of the "exhale gas" called carbon dioxide too quickly. Getting carbon dioxide out of your body too quickly causes your body to lose necessary acid. These chemical changes might cause your child to feel dizzy, cause him to feel as if he can't catch his breath or is choking, and cause his fingers or lips to tingle or even become numb.

Blowing Up a Balloon

The following breathing exercise should help your child feel more in control, allow him to get rid of the "funny feelings," and help him feel more relaxed.

Directions:
1. Have your child breathe into a paper bag for about 30 seconds with very slow, long exhalations.
2. If your child is anxious and has difficulty concentrating, suggest that he imagine a balloon that needs to be blown up.
3. Ask him to slowly start blowing and to imagine himself blowing up that big balloon.
4. Suggest that as he blows up the balloon, he notice its size, color, and shape, and whether there is any writing or pictures on the balloon.

After a few moments, let your child rest, and then repeat the procedure until he feels more relaxed and his breathing pattern has returned to normal. The exercise above is a good one to use during an acute pain or panic attack when there isn't much time to get your child's breathing under control.

Focused Breathing

The breathing exercise below requires a little more planning and time but is excellent for relaxing a child with chronic pain. You can practice this technique with your child, prompting her to take the next step, until she can do it on her own. Or you can read the instructions aloud into a tape recorder, very slowly, with pauses before each item. Then she can play the tape recorder as she carries out the exercise. Try this relaxation technique for at least 20 minutes a day. It is best to do the exercise with your child before the pain becomes too severe.

Directions:

1. Find a quiet room where you can get into a comfortable position to relax. The room should be fairly warm. When you become deeply relaxed, your body temperature drops and you can feel cold.
2. Close the door and tell other family members that you will need to be left alone for the next half hour (or as long as you would like). Put up a "do not disturb" sign, if you think that will help.
3. If the intent is to use this technique to go to sleep, do this exercise lying in bed ready for sleep.
4. If the intent is to use this technique to relax but not sleep, this exercise should be done sitting up, either sitting on the floor while leaning against a wall to support your back or sitting in a straight-backed chair. Your arms can drop comfortably in your lap.
5. Your eyes are closed.
6. Your arms and legs should not be crossed. This might cut off circulation and cause numbness and tingling.
7. Breathe in deeply and exhale slowly as though you were whistling. Do this slowly three times.
8. Count in your mind as you breathe out and see if you can get to a higher number each time that you breathe out (allowing yourself to breathe just a bit more slowly each time you breathe out).
9. Notice your body beginning to feel more relaxed with each breath out.
10. After three nice long breaths, you should begin to notice that tension in your body is moving through your body and out through your breath as you exhale.
11. Notice your body becoming heavy and limp, as if it were too much effort to even think about moving it. Or, conversely, you

may notice your body feeling weightless, or comfortably warm, as if you were floating in warm water.

12. You should notice that your breathing is nice and slow. At the end of your breath in, pause for a moment. Then, let the breath out again, nice and slow. Continue breathing in this way for a few minutes.

13. Notice your breath pushing down gently on your diaphragm. As this happens, you might notice your stomach begin to rise with each breath in. This is called "diaphragmatic breathing" and is the type of breathing that allows the most air into the lungs, with the least effort. (You can imagine your chest is an accordion, moving up and down as you breathe.)

14. As you practice this breathing exercise, your brain will learn how to change to diaphragmatic breathing and your diaphragm muscles will get stronger and stronger. This will bring more air into the lungs and you will begin to feel more and more refreshed at the end of the day, rather than fatigued.

15. To end the breathing exercise, you should first go back to breathing normally and effortlessly. Then focus on taking three purposeful long breaths by extending the exhalation nice and slow.

16. If you are in bed lying down and are using this technique to fall asleep, you may have fallen asleep somewhere in the middle of this exercise. If you have, this is fine. If you do this every night, your brain will learn to make the connections that indicate that it is time to fall asleep.

MUSCLE RELAXATION TECHNIQUES

Chronic pain can cause children to tense their muscles and even to hold their body in abnormal ways to protect themselves from stretching or injuring the painful body part. However, pain in one body area can create pain in another area because of muscle tension. This set of muscle relaxation exercises is meant to encourage muscles that are already tense to relax, prevent the buildup of stress in the muscles, and prevent muscle-related pain from developing. Again, you might want to first read these exercises to yourself and then read them into a tape recorder very slowly to record them.

Progressive Muscle Relaxation Exercise

Directions:
1. Allow yourself to be in a quiet place.
2. If you are doing this exercise to help you sleep, it is best to do this in your bed just before you are ready to go to sleep. For relaxation but not sleep, it is best to do this in a comfortable chair upright or in a recliner chair.
3. Take three slow deep breaths and then just continue to breathe normally. Notice your breathing.
4. You will begin to feel tension in your body flowing through your body and out through your breath. Notice energy from the air coming into your body through your lungs when you breathe in and feel it flow to the parts of your body where you need the most energy.
5. As you continue to breathe normally, focus your attention on your big toe on your right foot. With each breath out, notice that toe relaxing and feel its warmth as the circulation increases and more warm blood begins to flow through it.
6. Notice the relaxation beginning to spread to the big toe on your left foot, and notice that toe begin to feel relaxed and warm.
7. Notice the relaxation spreading in turn to each of the next toes on both feet—first, the toe next to the big toes, and then the next toe, and so on, until all of the toes on both feet feel relaxed, warm, and comfortable.

8. Notice the relaxation beginning to spread up to the top of your feet and under to the soles of your feet . . . spreading upward to your ankles, your calves, and shins, and up and around to your entire thighs. . . . Your feet might begin to feel so heavy that they can't even think about moving. They can just stay there and relax.

9. Now notice, with each breath out, as this wave of relaxation continues to move up your body . . . to your buttocks . . . lower back . . . and around to your pelvis. . . . You might notice your body feel as if it is sinking deeper into your bed or chair. Allow the feeling to flow in that direction, but whatever you feel is fine . . . just notice it.

10. As the wave of relaxation continues to move up your back and around to your belly, notice how your abdomen and back muscles feel when they begin to relax. This is a different feeling . . . warm . . . relaxation spreading up your body to your upper back and chest . . . to your shoulders and the area between your shoulder blades . . . around to your neck . . . front . . . sides . . . back of your neck.

11. Feel the relaxation spreading up into your head . . . the back of your head . . . sides . . . top . . . forehead . . . eyebrows . . . eyes. If they haven't closed by now, they may just want to close because the lids might feel too relaxed to be able to stay open . . . but whatever happens is fine.

12. Notice the relaxation spreading down your face to your cheeks . . . your nose . . . the area above your lip . . . your lips . . . your chin . . . around to your ears.

13. Now take a moment to enjoy the feeling of deep relaxation. . . . Feel yourself becoming more and more deeply relaxed with each breath out. . . . Allow your body to become as deeply relaxed as you would like to be and spend a few moments noticing how good it feels to be relaxed.

As you notice this feeling of relaxation, your brain will record it. This will become a new memory that can be called on when you need it. Each time you practice this relaxation exercise, that memory will become stronger and stronger. In time, you will need to take just three deep breaths and your brain will know exactly what to do. You will find yourself automatically going into a deep state of relaxation. You might find this happening even when you are busy doing other things. That is, you no longer will need to go through this exercise.

Muscle Relaxation/Muscle Contraction Exercise

Some people have a difficult time knowing what it feels like to have a muscle relax, especially people who have been in pain for a while. Chronically tense muscles use up energy when they are contracted. When you learn how to relax muscles, you free up energy so that you feel less tired and have the strength to get better. The exercise below will help you to feel the difference between muscle tension and muscle relaxation. It may be practiced on its own or in preparation for the progressive relaxation exercise described above.

Directions:

1. To begin, lie in your bed or sit in a comfortable chair, as above, depending on whether you are using this technique to help you (or your child) sleep or to relax and become energized.
2. Begin by taking three deep breaths as in the previous exercise, breathing out very slowly so that any tension in your body flows out of your body through your breath out and oxygen flows into your body with each breath in.
3. Contract your toes first by bending them down and squeezing as hard as you can and then just let them relax for a moment while you take two slow breaths.
4. Next, contract your ankles by bending your feet forward firmly

for as long as you can and then bending them back upward firmly toward your shins for as long as you can. Then allow your feet to relax while you take two very slow, deep breaths. Also take a moment to notice how relaxed your feet feel when they no longer have to do anything . . . just relax.

5. Contract the muscles of your legs. If you are sitting, you can do this by stretching your legs out straight in front of you and holding them as long and straight as you can until it takes too much effort to keep them there, and then you can let them go and just allow them to feel heavy and relaxed. If you are in bed, you can bend your knees and bring your knees to your chest if you can or bend them as much as you can and hold that position for as long as you can until it takes too much effort to continue, and then allow them to drop and become straight again, heavy, and relaxed. Again, when you are finished, take two very slow, deep breaths and just notice how relaxed your whole body is beginning to feel.

6. Next, if you are sitting in a chair, bend your upper body down toward your lap or below your knees if you are able to and hold that position. Keep pushing your upper body down . . . down . . . until it takes too much effort to keep it there. Then come back up and allow your whole body to sink deeply into the chair and relax. Again, take two very slow deep breaths and allow your body to just be without having to do anything during this time.

   If you are in bed doing this exercise, take three deep breaths and fill your lungs as your chest expands. Hold each breath for as long as you can before you slowly let out each breath. Notice your chest muscles beginning to relax as you breathe out each time. Again, take two very slow, deep breaths and allow your body to just be without having to do anything during this time.

7. Now expand your chest forward while you bring your shoulders back as close together as you can get them, making as deep a fold

between your shoulder blades as you can. Also, bring your shoulders downward. They should not be up by your ears. Hold this position for as long as your can, until it takes too much effort, and then release the pose. Again, take two very slow, deep breaths and allow your body to relax without having to do anything during this time.

8. Bend your arms by bringing your hands up to your shoulders, with your palms facing your shoulders, and squeeze your arms in that position for as long as you can until it takes too much effort. Then drop your arms at your sides and allow them to relax while you take two slow, deep breaths.

9. Now stretch your arms up as high as you can (if you are in bed, you can stretch them upward toward the ceiling) and keep your hands fully open, palms facing each other, and your fingers outstretched wide apart. Keep your arms and hands that way until it takes too much effort. Then drop them at your side and allow them to relax while you take two slow, deep breaths.

10. Finally, bend your head forward to touch your chin to your chest as far as you can go, and hold it for as long as you can until it takes too much effort. Then bring your head back up to a normal position. Do the same to the right and to the left, by turning your head to one side as long and deeply as you can and then to the other side as long and deeply as you can. Then allow your head and neck to relax while you take two slow, deep breaths.

11. Take just a few moments to be still and notice your breath as it returns to normal breathing again. Notice how deeply relaxed, warm, and comfortable your body feels without having to do anything, and just relax for a few moments while you breathe.

As you do this exercise with your child, you can turn it into a game. For a young child, you might want to suggest that she name her toes. Then your child can decide when each one has had enough and is ready to relax. Or you might want to create a challenge for each muscle that is being contracted. For example, when your child bends over, you might want to see how far downward he can bend or how close he can get his chin to his chest. Spending the time with your child carrying out this exercise can be helpful in itself. Remember, these exercises work best for your child if you first learn them for yourself, even if you don't have a pain problem. These are healthy exercises to enhance feelings of well-being.

HYPNOTHERAPY/GUIDED IMAGERY TECHNIQUES

We use hypnotherapy in our clinic to affect pain perception by accessing the part of the brain that creates mental images or pictures. When you use this part of your brain, you are able to biologically change the pain perception circuitry. As you learn self-hypnosis, the first thing you might notice is that the pain begins to fade into the background; that is, the pain may be there, but it doesn't bother you. This is what happens when you take morphine or other opioids for your pain.

I will now take you through the steps for self-hypnosis. I start with induction exercises, which are meant to relax you and help you to tune out the environment around you. The next series of exercises are called deepening techniques. They are methods for helping you to get into a more deeply relaxed state. Practice these exercises for yourself, and then you can teach them to your child. I provide you with some alternative strategies to use with your child.

You also can use this technique to fall asleep or to help your child to fall asleep. However, in the beginning, it is best to practice self-hypnosis sitting in a comfortable chair. It is important, as with all of these exercises, to have undisturbed time to practice. To begin, allow yourself to be in a comfortable body position and take a few breaths.

Induction Techniques: Ways to Enter a Hypnotic State

Progressive Relaxation

Progressive relaxation is the exercise that is described above, under "Progressive Muscle Exercise." It is useful, especially for adults and adolescents, to help to relax and tune out the world around you. This is a good exercise if you or your child has a difficult time focusing.

Arm Levitation

Imagine a string around your wrist that is tied to a big helium balloon. Can you feel it tugging at your wrist as the wind wants to carry it up into the sky? Notice as the balloon starts floating upward, so that your arm feels as if it is being pulled upward by the balloon . . . up and up . . . higher and higher. . . . You might notice your arm rising with the balloon. As your arm begins to rise and continues rising and when it begins to feel like too much effort to keep your arm up in the air, you can cut the string so the balloon floats away, way, way up into the air. Your arm may want to drop back down into your lap; if it does, let it. When your hand touches your lap (or arm of the chair), that can be a signal for your whole body to become deeply relaxed and comfortable.

Finger Magnet

Fold your hands together in front of your face as close as you can, but far enough away so that you can still see your fingers. Now straighten the index (for children, you may say *pointer*) finger of each hand while you keep the rest of your hands folded together. Separate these fingers as far apart as you can while still keeping the rest of your hands folded. Now imagine that there is a magnet inside each of the index fingers pulling them closer and closer together. Keep trying to resist and keep them apart. You might notice that the magnet is getting stronger and stronger. In fact, it might become hard to keep them apart, as if they had a mind of their own. . . .

You might notice them moving very slowly closer and closer together . . . until they touch. When this happens, it can be a signal to your body to become deeply relaxed, and your hands can fall to your lap (or arms of the chair), which will be a signal to your body to become more relaxed.

Spot on the Wall

Pick a spot on the wall near the ceiling in front of you. Keep staring as hard as you can on that spot until you start to notice that it is more and more difficult to keep your eyelids open. Each time that you blink, it may be more difficult to keep your eyes open. When your eyes are too heavy to stay open, they may close on their own. When that happens, you may notice that your whole body is deeply relaxed.

Eye Roll

Roll your eyes as far up and back into your head as possible, as if you were looking at a spot that is up inside the top of your head. Keep looking up as high into your head as possible, until it is no longer possible to continue. Let your eyeballs release, and that can be a signal for your eyes to close and for your body to become deeply relaxed. *(Do not practice this technique with contact lenses on!)*

Heavy Rock

Extend your arm with your palm facing up. Now imagine that someone is placing a heavy rock into your hand. Continue to hold that heavy rock up in the air for as long as you can until you notice the rock becoming very heavy and bearing down on your hand, making your arm feel so heavy and tired that it begins to fall downward . . . slowly . . . going down . . . down . . . heavier and heavier . . . until it feels too heavy and takes too much effort to continue to hold up the rock. When your arm feels too heavy to continue to hold the rock, your palm can turn over and let the rock go. When this happens, your arm may want to drop down to your lap (or arm of the chair). Let this be a signal for your whole body to become deeply relaxed and comfortable.

Painting

I learned the painting technique from a patient of mine. (Thank you, Tonya!) She had difficulty focusing on her breathing because that made her more anxious. She was in a wheelchair and had total body pain, so that even moving her arms was painful. She loved art and came up with this hypnotic induction technique. You can do this exercise with your eyes open or closed. Tonya says she initially did it with her eyes open and later closed them when she could do it by herself without any help.

Imagine that you are getting ready to paint. You can imagine a large white wall to paint on or a large canvas. . . . Before you begin, get all of your paints ready. Line up as many cans of paint colors as you want and in whatever order you want. Also bring as many different paintbrushes as you would like. When you are ready, you can dip one of your paintbrushes into the bucket. Notice whether the paint is watery and thin like painting with watercolors or really thick so that the paint may drip down the wall/canvas when you paint. Feel the paintbrush applying the paint to the wall/canvas . . . feel the broad strokes across . . . up and down . . . diagonally . . . circular . . . paint over other paint. . . . Just notice how good it feels to paint freely. When you have painted as much as you want, notice your mind leaving the paint and going to your favorite place.

Deepening Techniques

These exercises are meant to follow a hypnotic induction but may not be needed if your child is already in a trance or deep state of relaxation.

Stairs

Imagine you are at the top of a flight of stairs and there is a nice, thick, wooden banister to hold on to. Take hold of the banister and first take a few moments to feel the smooth wood of the carved banister. When you are ready, you can begin to go down the stairs. You might notice that there are 10 steps, for example. Breathe in deeply, and with each breath out, go down another stair. Notice that your body begins to feel more and more relaxed as you go down the stairs . . . step 9 and then 8 and 7. . . . With each breath and with each step, you feel your body become more deeply relaxed. . . . When you reach the bottom, you can find yourself in your favorite place.

Elevator

Imagine that you are in an elevator on the tenth floor. When you are ready, the doors will close. Notice the numbers above the door—the number *10* is lit up now. When you are ready, push the button to go down to the first floor . . . and you will feel the elevator start to go down. . . . With each breath out, notice the next lower number light up as the elevator goes down and down . . . *9* . . . *8* . . . *7*. . . . Feel yourself becoming more and more relaxed as each lower number is lit up . . . as you feel the elevator going down and down. . . . You can feel more and more relaxed . . . until you get to the first floor and the number *1* is lit up . . . and the doors open and you find yourself in your favorite place.

Favorite Place

Once you have attained a state of deep relaxation, you should find yourself in your favorite place. This place might be somewhere that you have been before . . . or somewhere that you would like to go . . . or maybe even at your home in your bed or room. Wherever you go is fine. The point of having a favorite place is to develop somewhere to "go" to feel safe and comfortable. This is especially important for children with chronic pain because they often feel off balance and uncomfortable. Feeling good and having positive emotions can help in the healing process, and deep relaxation also helps reduce the stress response in the body during pain.

One girl who had been in a wheelchair for two years because of total body pain was too anxious to picture herself dancing in her favorite place (she used to dance before developing her chronic pain problem), so she imagined herself at the dance studio watching herself dance, and over time, when she was ready, the watching gradually merged into the experiencing. In this way, the favorite place can also be used by a child to learn coping skills and to try a feared activity in small increments.

Directions:

1. Take a few moments to *really be there*! Notice the temperature . . . notice if the sun is out and if it feels warm . . . notice the warmth of the sun on your head and cheeks and shoulders. Just take a few moments to let that warm energy from the sun fill your body and refresh it. There might be a cool breeze. If so, you can notice the breeze feeling cool on your cheeks and lips. You might even hear the leaves in the trees rustle with the cool breeze. Take a few moments to look around you and notice the colors and whether you are by yourself or if anyone else is there with you—maybe your pet. Listen closely for any sounds . . . those that are close and those that are far in the distance. You might even notice what you are wearing and the texture of the ground beneath your feet if you are standing . . . maybe it is warm, dry sand or wet, squishy grass.

2. Notice how good it feels to be there and how good it feels to be relaxed and comfortable. You can be there for a while if you want.

Some younger children need extra help. For example, you might prompt them by asking them questions such as: *Are you at home in the room where your TV is? Let me know when you are there. Okay. Now turn on the TV. . . . What do you see on the TV? . . . What is happening? Is the sound up loud enough? Do you want to turn up the sound louder? . . . Tell me what you are watching and what is happening.*

Another way of helping a young child find a favorite place is to ask him about a favorite pet: *Are you with Tipper? Is Tipper on your lap or curled up next to you? Is his fur soft and warm? Doesn't it feel good to be cuddling with Tipper?*

Though *your* favorite place might be a relaxing, quiet environment such as the beach, often children want what is fun, and this might mean being active. For example, your child might want to be playing soccer. If this is the case, you'll tailor your prompts accordingly: *Notice yourself on the soccer field with your team . . . in your uniform. . . . Is it cool? Is the sun out? Oh, look—the ball is coming your way. . . . Do you have it? Wow! Did you just make that goal? Listen to your team shouting and jumping up and down for joy! "Great job!"*

Central Sensory Control Station

The goal of this technique is to help your child to gain control over and alter sensations that are painful in certain parts of the body. You can use a tape recording to begin. You can help your child with the exercise after you practice it and feel comfortable. The goal is for your child to practice this exercise and eventually commit it to memory. (There are many ways to do this technique; this description is just one of them.)

Directions:

1. Now that you are in your favorite place (or watching TV or playing ball or riding your bike); part of you can go to a different part of your brain, but the rest of you can continue being in your favorite place and enjoying being there. In this other part of your brain, look around and find the central control station for sensations or feeling. This might look like what a pilot might see at the front of a plane—lots of knobs and levers and switches and colored lights— but it might look like anything. . . . When you find it, just notice

it. . . . Now find the switch that controls the feeling to your [belly, head, or whatever body part has been hurting]. . . . Notice that it is not just an "on or off" switch but a dimmer switch. That means that you have control . . . you can turn it down as much or as little as you like. . . . so that only as much of the feelings from your belly (head, etc.) travels to your brain as you would like. . . . If you turned it all the way down, your belly (head, etc) would become numb with no feeling . . . so turn it down just as much as you need to. . . . As this is happening, you might notice changes in other parts of your body where you might have more feeling than before.

2. Your brain is now learning to change sensations or feelings in your body when you need to change them. Your brain will begin to get better and better at this like when you were really little and you were first learning the alphabet. After a while you just wrote without thinking about it. This is what your brain is learning to do now with feelings that you don't want to have in your body. It is learning to change them until they just go away or don't bother you as much anymore.

Posthypnotic Suggestion

The purpose of self-hypnosis or guided hypnosis (if you are doing it with your child) is to relax and leave your mind and body in a state of openness to suggestions, such as these:

- Now that you are enjoying yourself in your favorite place . . . and feeling so deeply relaxed and comfortable . . . just take a few moments to really be there. . . . Notice the feeling of deep relaxation so that your brain can absorb this memory.
- You have worked so hard and suffered so long that you deserve to take a few moments to just feel good.
- While you are relaxed, your brain is learning lots of new things to help you feel better. In fact, you may notice in the future that all you

need to do to become deeply relaxed is to take three slow, deep breaths and let them out slowly.

- You might notice that you sleep more deeply and restfully at night . . . a better sleep than you have had in a long time.

Exiting a Hypnotic State

It is good to help your child (or yourself, in self-hypnosis) to set a process for leaving the hypnotic state. Here is a guide for you to give your child, although you can develop your own strategy:

- In a few moments, you will be ready to return to the room and remain as comfortable as you want . . . continuing to be as deeply relaxed as you want, but with your mind alert and awake and your body feeling relaxed and full of energy.
- To do this, count backward from 10 to 1. Your body can remain as relaxed and comfortable as you want, but your mind will become more awake and alert as you count . . . with your eyes opening somewhere between 3 and 1. Take as long as you need in the next minute to count yourself out of hypnosis.

MINDFULNESS MEDITATION

Steven Weisman, M.D., the Jane B. Pettit Chair in Pain Management, Children's Hospital of Wisconsin, talks about mindful awareness and offers a meditative exercise:

"Mindful awareness can be a useful tool to help children and adolescents with chronic pain. Often, chronic pain invokes fear: fear of the unknown, fear that something is terribly wrong with one's body, fear of what school peers might think, and fear of losing control. Being able to cultivate mindful awareness of one's pain can help a child accept many of the feelings associated with the pain as well as give him insight into ways of actually controlling and regulating the pain.

"So how does one learn mindful awareness? I believe that this door is opened through learning the practice of mindfulness meditation. Long ago described by the Buddha as one of the means to overcome suffering, mindfulness meditation has been used extensively as a stress-reduction technique as well as in pain treatment plans. Traditionally, mindfulness meditation uses simple awareness of the breath to help focus the mind as it runs and jumps from thought to thought or sensation to sensation. It literally takes only one to two minutes to learn the basic fundamentals of mindfulness meditation.

"Simply find a comfortable, upright posture. If it is too uncomfortable to sit upright, lie down. The sitting posture tends to keep you from falling asleep. Some people find it helpful to sit on a cushion, but sitting in a chair or on a bench is perfectly fine. The arms can comfortably drop down from the shoulders and then the forearms can be placed on the thighs or in one's lap. You may keep your eyes open, gently gazing ahead, possibly at a spot on the floor or a wall. You might also choose to close your eyes. After a moment or two, check in with yourself so that you feel comfortable, and direct your attention to your breath. Feel the air as it moves through your nostrils or mouth. Feel the breath as it fills your abdomen. Feel the abdomen rise up and then deflate down. Focus your slow, comfortable breaths into the lower abdomen so that your breathing becomes regular and deep. As you do this, it is natural for your attention to wander onto other thoughts or feelings. As you become aware of these thoughts and feelings rising up, acknowledge that your mind has wandered, and then simply and gently, guide it back to your breath. Continue this for several minutes. If you notice some discomfort in your body due to your posture, then with awareness of the body, shift to a more acceptable position. Try this when you awaken in the morning, or when you have a few spare moments. Surely you can find a few moments to practice in the evening or even before going to bed.

Below is a simple breath poem to help guide the breath during sitting meditation.

Breathing in, I know I am breathing in. . . .

Breathing out, I know that I am breathing out.

Breathing in, I calm my body. . . . Breathing out, I smile.

Breathing in, I am aware of the present moment. . . .

Breathing out, I offer love to my body.

Breathing in, I calm my mind. . . . Breathing out, I am thankful to be alive.

Breathing in, I release my fears. . . . Breathing out, I release my thoughts.

Breathing in, I know I am breathing in. . . .

Breathing out, I know that I am breathing out.

Cultivating mindfulness can bring benefits beyond our expectations. It brings profound relaxation to the body and mind. Over time, with the practice of mindful awareness, many children will notice a reduction in their pain and other symptoms. Often the results are not obvious. But it is precisely the moving away from the need to have results that often contributes to a lessening of the child's suffering.

SLEEP

Is Your Child Getting Enough Sleep?

To find out whether your child is getting enough sleep, take note of the answers to the questions below. If you answer yes to several of these questions, the chances are that your child isn't getting enough quality sleep, especially if she has a chronic pain problem.

- Does your child have trouble falling asleep at night?
- Does she have problems staying asleep once she falls asleep? If she wakes up during the night, how often does she waken, and does she have trouble falling back asleep?
- Does she have difficulty getting up in the morning?
- Does she feel fatigued during the day and not rested?
- Does she have trouble establishing a routine before she goes to bed?
- Does she nap during the day?

- Does she take any medication for sleep? If so, does this medication make her feel groggy the next day?

How to Help Your Child Get a Better Night's Sleep

Sleep is a cornerstone of pain relief. Not getting enough restorative (refreshing, healing, deep) sleep can be devastating to a child's body. Children typically need more sleep than do adults. Children with chronic pain who are not getting sufficient restorative sleep have more difficulty learning how to cope because their brain does not learn as well when they are sleep-deprived. This may be especially true for adolescents, whose sleep cycle is often at odds with the requirements of the school system. The lack of restorative sleep at night creates a vicious cycle: Chronic pain can cause insufficient sleep, and insufficient sleep can maintain the pain.

The key to dealing with chronic pain is to know as much as you can about how well your child is functioning. If she isn't getting enough sleep, she probably isn't functioning as well as she could. Developing a plan and a strategy to, for example, make sure she gets a good night's sleep, is the first step. For example, if James has trouble sleeping at night, the answer isn't "What one thing can I do to get him to sleep" or, as I often hear, "Can you give him something to make him fall asleep?" If James is not falling asleep, let's review the possible reasons why he is not. Once you know the reason why, it is much easier to come up with a treatment plan. Take note of the following:

- What time is he eating dinner? (If he is eating a heavy meal right before he is supposed to go to sleep, the food may be interfering with his sleep.)
- Is he consuming caffeine products, such as soda, chocolate, or tea, before bed?
- What does he do after dinner and at night to get ready for bed? Does he watch TV or work on his computer or play video games?

(The more active he is, especially on the computer or with video games, the more aroused his nervous system will become and the harder it will be for him to fall asleep.)

- Does he watch TV, play computer games, and so on while in his bed? (The bed should be the place where he can read or listen to music and get ready to go to sleep, not a place for exciting activities at night.)

- Does he have a bedtime routine? (Developing routines is helpful, especially for the child who has sleep difficulty.)

- If he is young, perhaps younger than 13, do you spend any time with him at bedtime in his room so that bedtime is associated with pleasant parent-related activities (such as telling him a story; massaging his head, neck, and shoulders; or talking about things that happened during the day)?

- Is he sleeping in his bed or in your bed? (The goal is for him to sleep in his bed.)

- Does he have or need a night-light?

Once you've asked and answered these questions, you can start developing a strategy to help your child sleep better. This is the type of thinking that will help your child to cope better. The following are some good guides for sleeping, or good sleep hygiene:

- Set a schedule. Your child should go to bed at a set time each night and get up at the same time each morning. Many adolescents are sleep-deprived during the week with homework, late nights, and early mornings for school, and weekends are their catch-up time. However, for some children, weekend sleep patterns may make it more difficult to wake up early on Monday mornings. See what works best for your child.

- Don't lie in bed awake. If your child can't get to sleep, he shouldn't just lie in bed. Let him do something else, such as reading or listening to soft music, until he feels tired. The worry about trying to fall asleep can keep him awake.

- Exercise. Your child should exercise 20 to 30 minutes a day. Daily exercise will help her sleep, but it is best to exercise about five to six hours before going to bed, because exercising too close to bedtime can interfere with sleep.

- Sleep until sunlight. If possible, wake up with the sun, or use very bright lights in the morning. Sunlight helps the body's internal biological clock reset itself each day. It is often helpful for a child to get at least an hour of morning sunlight if he has problems falling asleep at night.

- Control the room temperature. Maintain a comfortable temperature in the bedroom. Room temperatures that are too hot or too cold can prevent your child from falling asleep or wake her up during the night.

- Avoid caffeine products. Your child should avoid drinks that contain caffeine, because it acts as a stimulant and will keep her awake.

- If the above steps do not help your child get restful sleep (or even if they do), teach him any of the relaxation techniques for use in bed: progressive relaxation, breathing exercises, self-hypnosis (see above).

- If your child is napping during the day, try to interrupt this pattern so that your child will be more tired at night.

- For younger children, setting up a bedtime routine with a parent is very helpful. For example, the last thing that your child might do before sleep is to listen as you to read him a story while he is in his bed, or relax as you massage his head and back. That is, develop some calming routine together that will be associated with relaxing.

GETTING THROUGH A BAD PAIN DAY

Stress can increase the amount of pain, reduce pain tolerance, and cause a pain relapse. The most common time for pain to relapse is the start of the school year. Other stresses can be related to family members (such as parents' marital discord, death of a pet, illness in a parent). A viral infection in your child can set off a bout of IBS symptoms or headaches. Lack of sufficient sleep, travel, or overdoing it with an activity on a weekend can also be causes. Some of these have relatively easy solutions: more rest, sleep, or the opportunity for your child to talk about what is bothering her. Others may not be so easy to solve. Try these steps:

1. Identify sources of stress and help your child learn how to deal with them.

2. Identify warning signs. New headaches, excessive fatigue, irritability, or moping can be warning signs of an impending relapse of chronic pain.

3. Develop a game plan. A game plan may include some of the following strategies:

   • Maintaining a normal schedule: Encourage your child to get out of the house and schedule plans with friends or go to school.

   • Helping your child seek distractions: Encourage him to read something he likes, watch a funny movie, call a friend, play video games or work on the computer, go outside to play, be with friends, or do something physically active.

   • Encouraging your child to relax: Relaxation quiets the CNS and can reduce pain.

4. Use medications wisely. Drugs are not the only answer to pain and shouldn't be the first tool that you use when your child begins to complain of pain or becomes irritable. If the first thing that you do when your child has pain is to reach for medications or tell him to take a pill, this "medication first" plan will train your child to turn to medications rather than himself when he is not feeling well.

5. Let your child know that you are confident he can get through this and that it will pass. If you show that you have confidence in him, he will learn to have confidence in himself.

THE ABCS OF GETTING GOOD CARE
FOR YOUR CHILD

- Find a doctor who listens.
- Ask your child's physician and the other clinicians to whom your child may be referred for treatment (e.g., physical therapist) if they have experience dealing with pain problems in children or adolescents.
- Find a doctor who believes that your child is in pain.
- Make sure that there is a treatment plan.
- Don't make the doctor king or queen. Doctors do not know everything. I am always learning something new from my patients, from reading scientific literature, and from discussions with other physicians and other clinicians. Your child's doctor should have the humility to admit when she doesn't know something and be willing to learn more about it and then get back to you to discuss it, or to refer your child to someone who is more familiar with your child's pain problem.
- Ask the physician to explain her diagnosis of the problem so that it makes sense to you. If you don't understand, tell the doctor and ask her to explain it again.
- Choose a doctor with whom you can have open communication (e-mail, phone calls, etc.), or set up a plan for how to best communicate.
- You need to be assured that your child's doctor is willing to communicate with the other doctors and clinicians who are caring for your child. You should not have to hear one diagnosis of your child's problem from the physician, another from the acupuncturist, and another from the chiropractor. Ask your child's doctor to talk with the other clinicians who are caring for your child so that they are all familiar with and up-to-date on your child's case.

- Seek out all resources. Get as much information as you can through books and the Internet. Use this information to raise questions with your child's physician. Being an informed parent is the best way to advocate for your child's care.

- Always consider complementary therapies, PT, psychotherapy, or family therapy, not just medications. With rare exceptions, medications alone do not work for most children with chronic pain.

- If you are dissatisfied with what your doctor has explained to you about your child's pain and/or the treatment plan doesn't make sense to you, then it is fine to get a second opinion.

- Doctors need to take children seriously. Your child's physician should not belittle or make fun of your child; this is different from having fun with your child and you during an evaluation.

- You should never continue with a doctor who talks down to you. Your job is not to massage his ego.

- Try to establish a method for contacting your child's doctor with nonurgent questions, such as through e-mail, or write down the questions to be addressed during a visit with your child's physician.

- Always ask about the side effects of a new medication, when you should stop giving that medication, or what to do if you observe side effects.

{ CHAPTER ELEVEN }

Answers to Parents' Questions

I have found the best way to give advice to your children is to find out what they want and then advise them to do it.

—HARRY S. TRUMAN

In this chapter, I answer specific questions that parents have asked over the years. The questions are organized into the following subject categories: When Your Child Can't Sleep, Helping Your Child Cope, Life at Home, When Your Child Relapses, Your Child's Doctor, Your Child's School.

WHEN YOUR CHILD CAN'T SLEEP

Parents of a child with chronic pain commonly worry whether their child is getting enough sleep. They are right to worry. Chronic pain can cause a child to lose sleep, and a lack of sleep can cause more pain—it's a vicious cycle. (For tips on helping your child get a better night's sleep, see Chapter 10, "Helping Your Child Cope with Chronic Pain," pages 232–234.)

Why is sleep so important for a child with chronic pain?

Deep sleep refreshes the body and mind, improves attitude, and restores the energy needed for physical activity and to fight off fatigue and stress. It also boosts the immune system, reducing the risk of illness. Long-term sleep deprivation may be one important factor in the *development* of chronic pain conditions in some children. Here are some other reasons why it's important for a child to get enough sleep:

- Lack of sleep can leave a child with chronic pain tired, in a poor mood, irritable, more easily frustrated, less able to concentrate, and less motivated to do things that might help in his physical and psychological recovery.
- Sleep loss can increase a child's perception of pain and sensitivity to pain sensations, further eroding sleep and increasing pain.
- Certain neurotransmitters and hormones thought to be critical to normal physical development and the repair of damaged tissue are released during sleep.
- At sleep onset there is a reduction in the release of stress hormones, such as cortisol, and during sleep there is a dampening of the effects of stress, such as chronic pain, on the immune system.

My daughter is always tired in the morning even if she has had a full night's sleep. Why is this?

This daytime fatigue may be related to the quality of the sleep that she is getting. Human sleep is a succession of five recurring stages: four non-REM stages and the REM (rapid eye movement) stage. She may not be getting enough deep sleep (stage 3 or 4, also called restorative sleep). If she spends most of the night in light stages of sleep (stage 1 or 2) or REM stage, she will not have enough restorative sleep and will feel tired throughout the day. REM sleep is marked by extensive physiological changes, such as accelerated breathing, increased brain activity, eye movement, and muscle relaxation. If she does not have enough deep sleep, then she will be less likely to cope with pain.

My son is able to sleep only a few hours a night because of muscle pain in his arms and legs. Which sleeping medications are safe for children?
First, try the techniques for better sleep in Chapter 10 ("Helping Your Child Cope with Chronic Pain"). You can also try melatonin (1 to 3 milligrams at night to restore circadian sleep rhythms, herbs such as valerian root (taken in capsule form about one hour before bedtime), and chamomile (manzanilla) tea. Magnesium (500 milligrams one or two times a day) can also be helpful for muscle cramps, although it can cause diarrhea if the dose is too high. If none of these help and he still needs a medication to sleep, one of the following can be used with the help of your child's physician: Desyrel (trazodone), Neurontin, Restoril, Remeron. Ambien can also be effective, but I tend to not use it because it is addictive, unlike the other medications. Medications that block deep stages of sleep, such as benzodiazepines (e.g., Ativan, Klonopin, Xanax, Valium), are useful only if his anxiety is so elevated that other antianxiety medications are not effective alone. Sometimes sleep problems can be the result of anxiety or depression. If so, then an SSRI (e.g., Zoloft or Celexa) and psychotherapy can be helpful to target these symptoms and restore deep sleep.

HELPING YOUR CHILD COPE

The primary goal in treating pediatric chronic or recurrent pain is to help children learn how to cope so that they can increase their functioning—participate in activities, go to school, sleep, and eat—so that eventually the pain will go away on its own. Many parents understandably want to make things "all better" for their child so that their child won't have to suffer, so they look for a magic pill. However, it is far better to help him learn how to get through a day of school, how to relax, or how to reconnect with his friends than to simply focus on a cure. Your child will begin to get better when he feels less anxiety about his pain and more self-reliant and in control. Many years ago, someone I know described a "good parent" as one who loves her child but can also teach her child how to become self-reliant and feel confident. This has stuck with me.

How do I step back and let my daughter help herself?

Here's an answer for you from one of my former patients. Beginning when she was nine years old Beth suffered from severe leg pain that was made worse by several knee surgeries. Today, at the age of 18, she credits her parents with helping her get better by letting her do things for herself:

• • •

> As much as it was painful for my mom (she was with me at home during the day), she did the right things. If I was at school and I'd call home and want her to come get me, she wouldn't come get me or she wouldn't answer the phone. It sounds absolutely horrible, and it would infuriate me at the time, but she had to let go. I was forced to do things on my own, and it helped me get through the recovery stage. There is a point where you're in so much pain and it's easy to have everything done for you. But this way, I was forced to recover.

• • •

Beth's mom wasn't always this good at letting go; she had to learn. I remember Beth's mom pushing Beth in her wheelchair to a visit in my office, and Beth was happy to let her mom do this, even though she was quite capable of wheeling herself. Sometimes, it took not only reminding Beth's mom that she didn't have to wheel her but actually holding her back physically while Beth wheeled herself. We all laughed about it later, but it was a powerful reminder. For a child, there is something very powerful about surviving a day at school even though she is in pain. She learns that the pain will not kill her and that she has the strength and ability to overcome it. Many parents, especially mothers, have to unlearn the instinctual urge to take over and do everything, so that the child has the opportunity to help herself.

Might an active child still be in pain?

Children are extremely resilient, and being active in the face of chronic and even acute pain is often a sign of effective coping. In fact, for any pain condition, remaining active even while in pain can actually help get rid of the pain over time. This is why the primary focus in chronic pain is function first and elimination of pain second.

Just because a child is able to cope with his pain doesn't mean it doesn't exist. In public arenas such as sports or school, children learn to control their reaction to acute pain because they are motivated to do so, usually out of a desire to fit in and do what their classmates are doing. Children with chronic pain feel a sense of control and mastery over the pain when they are able to function in spite of it. Continuing to function also increases circulation to muscles and releases brain endorphins that are important in pain control.

Can dietary changes help IBS pain?

IBS is primarily a brain–gut nervous system problem in which the nerve signaling has become dysregulated. The resulting increased sensitivity in the intestine leads to belly pain and secondary gut motor problems, including diarrhea, constipation, or both, as well as bloating, nausea, and sometimes vomiting. For true IBS, diet generally does not make a difference. However, there is some preliminary evidence that a low-fat diet may be helpful in reducing some of the symptoms of IBS. I would recommend a "lowish"-fat diet. Children need some fat in their diet for brain growth, but they should get the "good" fats from foods such as salmon and avocadoes rather than the "bad" saturated fats found in many snack foods. Also, taking one or two peppermint oil geltabs (found in health food stores) before meals has been found to reduce pain for some children.

Why is my son's pain worse in the evening?

Pain typically increases in the evening for most people. This happens because (1) there are fewer distractions than in the daytime, (2) exhaustion from the day's activities can reduce effective coping, and (3) fears about not being able to sleep can increase pain signals. Also, if evening is a time when the entire family is present, this might be the only time when your son can let everyone know how much he is suffering. I suggest some focused time in the evening spent on positive activities, such as reading together or talking, as well as developing a routine in the evening. (See Chapter 10, "Helping Your Child Cope with Chronic Pain," for strategies.)

LIFE AT HOME

When a child develops a chronic or recurrent pain problem, there is suddenly a new member of the family: The Pain. Nobody wants this new family member, but it has moved in and made itself quite comfortable as the center of attention. This new family member can start dictating what the family can and cannot do, such as going out to dinner or taking vacations. You may find yourself spending more and more time taking care of it, which can take its toll on your family life. Everything can suffer—your sleep, work, marriage, and your relationship with your children.

I am finding myself getting very angry at and frustrated with my son. Later I feel guilty. Is this normal? What can I do?

This is absolutely normal. Many parents (typically—but not always—moms) feel responsible and guilty for their child's pain problem. You see your child suffering with pain and feel helpless to make it better. But your child's pain is not your fault. Having a child with chronic pain can leave you feeling tired, frustrated, and helpless. All of these feelings can lead to irritability, anxiety, and anger, which may cause you to lash out at your son for "just lying around moaning" and not doing anything. You then feel guilty about being angry.

To prevent these conflicts, it is helpful for you to take care of yourself. Notice if you are becoming stressed and treat yourself to something nourishing and relaxing. Remember what flight attendants say when reviewing safety instructions on the plane just before takeoff: "Adjust your own oxygen mask before helping your child with his." You can't help your child if you are also stressed. Practice the relaxation techniques in this book yourself. Talk about your feelings with your spouse or partner, friends, or a therapist. Recognizing and talking about how you feel is the first step in letting go of those feelings. It is fine to apologize to your son later if you think that your behavior toward him was not fair or was too harsh. He will not blame you for the rest of his life. If he is angry for a while, that is fine. Anger is an important emotion that is better expressed and released than held on to until your body reacts.

When my 10-year-old son is in terrible pain, he acts out and won't listen to me. How do I set limits for him and still be empathetic?
If by *acts out* you mean that he curses you, throws things, or commits other destructive acts, then your child is out of control and you need to set limits so that he doesn't injure himself or anyone else. If this destructive behavior happens when he is having a bad pain episode, then you need to inform him that this is unacceptable behavior, help him find an acceptable alternative for letting out his frustration, provide consequences (removal of privileges) if he continues with this destructive behavior after being informed, and provide incentives for changing his behavior and coping better.

The best way to help him is to set up strategies together to prevent this behavior: coping techniques, a behavioral incentive plan, or professional help (which could include psychotherapy, yoga, hypnotherapy, or other clinical help). The problem may also be a family systems problem, in which his behavior serves some function in the family that no one yet recognizes. For example, if you and your spouse or partner are having difficulties, such behavior on the part of your son might be his way of diverting your attention from each other and onto him—his way of trying to help the two of you. In this case, family or couples therapy might be helpful.

My daughter's CRPS requires a lot of family attention. I feel it is causing problems for my other children. What can I do?

It will be helpful for you to consider how much individual time you give not only to your daughter with CRPS but to each of your children. Each will need some of your individual, undivided attention, whether that means taking a walk together, reading a story at night, or some other activity. Your other children may complain more about their aches and pains as a way to subtly tell you that they are feeling left out and jealous of the attention their sister receives. Their resentment might also cause them to act out behaviorally or, conversely, to become more withdrawn.

Resentment also can build in relation to chores. Is she exempt from chores completely because of her pain? Are they taking her share as well as theirs? I do not advise either situation. All children should have some chores to do if they are living at home. Your daughter with CRPS should have chores that are reasonable to expect of her. This will then be one area where the other children won't begin to resent their sister. And it will help your daughter not to feel different from everyone else (even if she complains).

Talk with your children about their feelings. Allow them to express jealousy, anger, resentment, or whatever feelings they have toward one another, including your daughter with CRPS, because she will likely also have feelings about her siblings. It is important to listen to your children, empathize, and avoid trying to reason with them. Just letting them know that you understand and also providing some individual time with each of your children will go a long way toward reducing unwanted behaviors. If this approach doesn't work, you may need to seek family therapy so that you do not allow the pain to take over.

One day during the last week of school, Brooke came home from school early with a stomachache she said was the worst she'd had since summer. That evening she was in tears because two friends were moving away and two were going on to high school. I am sure these issues are connected to her pain. Am I right? What can I do?

You are likely right about the connection. Talking can always be helpful. Wondering out loud to Brooke about what she may be feeling can be a very useful way to bring the issues out in the open. For example, you might say: "How sad you must feel with two friends moving and two leaving your school. That is a loss. I would feel sad if they were my friends and I was in your situation. I certainly would not be surprised if you had stomach pains because your body just needed to let out stress and sadness."

Then I would encourage her to talk more about her feelings. Even if she denies feeling sad and just focuses on the pain, she still will have heard the connection you made between her friends moving, sad feelings, and her stomach pains. She may need time to figure this out for herself. She also may benefit from some relaxation strategies with your help to reduce the pain (see Chapter 10, "Helping Your Child Cope with Chronic Pain").

These treatment options are taking a toll on my finances. What can I do?

Some parents say that they can't afford hypnotherapy, biofeedback, yoga, or family therapy for their child, yet they take expensive vacations and eat out in restaurants often. In such cases, it is a matter of setting priorities: Will they focus on family luxuries or on their child's health and well-being? However, the reality is that many of the most effective chronic pain treatments are not covered by insurance and paying for them is prohibitive for many families. If this is the case for your family, you may have to make a choice and focus on one therapy, possibly working out a payment plan with the clinician.

I know families who have taken out loans to pay for a therapy that wasn't covered by insurance because it was the only thing that made their child's pain better. You might seek help from foundations or your place of worship. It is also helpful to check the Web site of the university nearest to you to see if they have any open research studies that offer what you want, because the treatment in that case is free. Also, some graduate students or psychology interns do free cognitive testing or psychotherapy in student clinics, with supervision from licensed psychologists. Similarly, massage and acupuncture schools tend to have lower fees, and centers of learning, such as Iyengar yoga institutes and Zen Buddhism or Vipassana meditation centers, may provide low-cost yoga or meditation instruction.

My husband is not engaging with our son. What can I do?
First, examine your own behavior. Is your husband not engaging because you are leaving him little room to engage? Seek his advice on helping your son with his pain. There are plenty of issues to discuss, such as how to help your son become more physically active, how to develop a plan for him to return to school, how to help him learn tools for coping with pain. Develop strategies together regarding who will help your son with what. For example, ask your husband to take a walk with your son, shoot hoops, or distract him with a board or computer game. Your husband needs to set a good example for your son about how to cope and function in the face of stress. And you need his help because he is the best same-sex role model your son has.

WHEN YOUR CHILD RELAPSES

One of the worst experiences for families of children with chronic pain is when a child relapses after a period of being pain free and back to a normal life. Relapses can be more demoralizing than the original pain. Most children with chronic pain remain vulnerable to pain even after they have gotten better, and even if your child has mastered self-soothing techniques (e.g., yoga, cognitive-behavioral strategies, self-hypnosis, biofeedback), he may still be at risk for a relapse. An infection, injury, or stress at school or at home can trigger a relapse. For this reason, it is important that a child be taught to identify signs of a problem, such as headaches that become more frequent or last a bit longer, or continued pain after the stomach flu when everyone else in the family who has had the flu feels better. If he has learned coping strategies, he can employ these before the relapsed pain gets out of control. He might also need some refresher sessions with the clinician who helped him the first time.

My daughter had been pretty much free of the pain from fibromyalgia for more than a year. Then one day, she was back where she had started. What did we do wrong? How do we handle her relapse?

Many of the same strategies that applied the first time apply the next time. First, assess what is going on. Why was there a recurrence of the pain problem this time? Did your daughter have the flu, a fight at school, a problem with a particular class? Something usually sets off the nervous system again, and it is helpful to think this through together with your daughter. Sometimes a transition—for example, from middle school to high school, a move to a different neighborhood, or a friend moving away—can be enough to trigger a relapse. Address as many of the possible factors as you can, one by one. Be sure also to consider factors that you didn't the first time.

The fact that your child relapsed doesn't mean that you did anything wrong. Don't give up. If she got through it once, that means that she can do it again—and each time, it should get a bit easier. One caveat: If you relied solely on medication the first time and your child hasn't learned coping skills, then she is at higher risk for developing a recurrence of the pain problem. This is why I always encourage families to help their child learn at least one active coping strategy.

The family of a 15-year-old patient of mine learned about relapses the hard way. The family had worked incredibly hard for several years to help their son who had been suffering from chronic pain due to fibromyalgia. They had weaned him off Demerol, he learned coping strategies, and they underwent family therapy to learn more positive ways to interact with one another. They were so successful that he was back in school full-time, on the school football team, and had a full academic and social life. Then, about two years later, his mother recalls:

* * *

> I was pretty naive when he relapsed. The first time Paul went into the hospital for his pain rehabilitation program, he had to have three or four shots of Demerol a day. When he left after the eight weeks, he was on no pain medication whatsoever, and for the next two years, he never took anything stronger than an ibuprofen . . . even when he had football injuries. So I felt like the techniques that he had were going to serve him and serve him well for the rest of his life. At the two-year mark, he wasn't pain free, but it wasn't anything that impacted his life in any way. It was like normal life. The first time, he had been out of school for a whole year and his pain was so horrible, and so excruciating.
>
> So when he started to get headaches, his dad and I were very much telling him you need to do relaxation techniques and exercise. It was basically just . . . expecting Paul to have the same results [as before]. Well, Paul was 15½ years old at this point, and so not only was there normal 15-year-old stuff with school and girlfriend, there was a great deal of anxiety as a normal 15-year-old, in addition to Paul's pain anxiety disorder and fibromyalgia. So Paul's anxiety drove his pain, his pain drove his anxiety, and his anxiety drove his pain. It made a loop. And for some reason, this time, Paul was not able to go in and close down the pain gates in his brain. His anxiety level was so high. His central nervous system was so aroused and irritated that he was just not able to do it. He got worse and worse. We were thinking, *Paul's just not applying himself enough*.

* * *

But Paul did get better. Many families feel devastated—as in "Oh, no! Here we go again!"—if their child's pain problem relapses. But this time you are all smarter: You know more about your child's neurology, you know more about chronic pain, and you know more about different coping strategies. Seek help if the old plan needs a tune-up.

YOUR CHILD'S DOCTOR

To advocate for your child, you need to know how to educate and negotiate with your child's doctor and other clinicians if you think that they don't understand the problem or are not approaching it with treatment that is helpful. Appendix B of this book is a list of pediatric pain programs around the United States, Canada, and elsewhere to which you can turn for expert advice in pediatric chronic pain, including specialty clinics for functional bowel disorders.

My son sees a doctor several times a week for his CRPS. I feel that the doctor does not respect my opinion, and he does not explain my son's condition to me so that I can understand. What can I do?

First, why is your child seeing a doctor "several times a week" for CRPS? What is he doing during those visits? Your son would do far better in PT several times a week after school. If your doctor won't answer your or your son's questions and you feel that he is discounting or ignoring your input, is doing things that you disagree with, or is not discussing his treatment approaches to your satisfaction, then I would say that you should find a new doctor. I believe that a key element in the healing process is the relationship among you, your child, your child's physician (or the coordinator of your child's pain management plan), and other treating clinicians. Ideally, this relationship is based on mutual respect and trust and a sense that you are working together to relieve your child's pain.

I often become overwhelmed in my child's doctor's office and forget what to ask. Are there some questions I should be sure to ask the doctor?

I think it is helpful to talk with your child and with your spouse or partner in advance of the appointment, to make sure you all understand the diagnosis and treatment plan. Come up with questions you want answered and *write them down*. If you are afraid that you won't remember what the doctor said in response to your questions, bring a tape recorder to the appointment so you can listen to her responses at your leisure and rewind the tape if you didn't understand something the first time you played it.

David Fleisher, M.D., professor of pediatrics at the University of Missouri and an expert in pediatric functional gastroenterology, offers the following advice: "Be sure your doctor listens to you and doesn't rush you. And, having heard your history and listened to your concerns, your doctor should be expected to convey the *three essential communications* that satisfy your intellectual and emotional needs":

1. **Clarity:**
   - What's the diagnosis or likely diagnosis?
   - What goes on in my child's body that causes the pain?
   - Is it safe or dangerous?
   - What can be done about it, and which tests and treatments will likely not be helpful and can be dispensed with?
   - What's the outlook? Is it something that can be cured quickly, or will it take time and effort?
2. **Effective reassurance:** Reassurance becomes effective when it speaks to and relieves your spoken and also hidden fears that motivated you to seek help for your child.
3. **The offer of continuity and accessibility:** The doctor has to be willing to own the problem with you until it is over. This gives you the backup you need to stay on course and be able to have expectations of your child to keep up with her daily activities and to avoid becoming an invalid.

The doctors have tried everything. What next?

If *everything* means that they've prescribed many medications and procedures and "nothing is working," then you need to explore any or several of the nondrug, complementary therapies, including hypnotherapy, biofeedback, acupuncture, massage therapy, energy therapies, art therapy, and therapeutic yoga, as well as PT and psychological therapy. You can coordinate your child's care by yourself, but it would be best if you could find a pediatric pain specialist to coordinate your child's pain management plan, unless your child's primary care physician is willing to do this and contact a pediatric pain specialist for help as needed.

My daughter has severe abdominal pain. Are all the tests really necessary?

In medical school, I learned that if you take the time to carry out a complete history and physical examination, you should have a pretty good idea of what is causing the problem without conducting a battery of tests. Sometimes tests are needed to confirm the suspected problem, such as brain MRI for a child with severe, protracted headaches. However, the tests should be limited to confirm what the history and examination findings already point to. Using tests to rule out illnesses or diseases simply because a doctor doesn't know what else to do is bad medicine.

Paul Hyman, M.D., a good friend and head of pediatric gastroenterology at the University of Kansas Medical Center, taught me the fine art of examining a belly in a child with belly pain without resorting to lots of tests and medical procedures. For example, I learned that belly pain in a child with IBS could be related to contracted and painful rectus abdomini muscles that are located in the middle of the belly. This is a cause of pain that may be overlooked if everyone is assuming that the intestines are causing the pain. Massage, therapeutic yoga, and PT can all relieve this kind of muscular-related belly pain.

YOUR CHILD'S SCHOOL

For thousands of children who suffer from chronic pain, typical child-hood stresses can be difficult hurdles. School, in particular, presents all kinds of social and learning pressures. Irregular school attendance is one of the biggest challenges. As the child begins to miss school, the pressure begins to mount until going to school begins to feel like an inconquerable obstacle. Other factors, such as learning and emotional disabilities and uneven cognitive development, can contribute to stress and pain. Social problems—whether or not they are related to the medical condition—or an unsympathetic teacher also can cause a child to avoid going to school. Rather than addressing these factors, the child might find it easier to make pain the culprit for these school absences.

I asked Caryn Freeman, a wonderful teacher and friend, to address some of the most important questions related to school that parents of children with chronic pain have asked over the years. Besides having a master's degree in educational psychology, Caryn has been teaching with the Los Angeles Unified School District since 1968. The questions and answers that follow will provide you with insights and ideas that you can use when dealing with your child's teachers, school administrators, and peers.

My son, Alex, is in tenth grade. He has chronic stomachaches that keep him out of school about one third of the semester. Although having a teacher come to our home once a week is an option, I would prefer that my son have a normal school experience. Is this possible?

[C. Freeman:] It is certainly possible if you choose the appropriate school and teachers for Alex. When it comes to students who need to be absent, certain private and public schools are much more flexible than others. The school should agree to give him credit if he successfully completes all of the work. You need to speak to an administrator at Alex's school. Explain Alex's situation honestly and find out how flexible the school is with regard to illness absences. Remember that school administrators legally have to make some accommodations for Alex. The Rehabilitation Act and the Individuals with Disabilities Education Act (IDEA) of 1990 guarantee access to school for children with chronic and handicapping conditions. Children with special health care needs must be integrated into the regular school setting, and schools must modify and adapt their environment and programs to accommodate these children.

It is important that you find an administrator (possibly the head counselor) who will work with you and your son to pick teachers and classes that will be the most flexible and accommodating. Given that the school and teachers are willing to cooperate, the way to ensure that Alex is successful and not overly stressed is to make sure he makes up the work and tests *on time*. Because Alex suffers from chronic pain rather than a debilitating illness (in which case homeschooling might be your only option), even when he is absent from school he can probably do some work during those times of the day when the pain subsides. In each class, Alex needs to have a friend (or a student picked by the teacher—possibly for extra-credit points) who can inform him *each day* of the classwork and homework Alex needs to do. If the classwork or homework involves papers that are passed out in class, the teacher should provide the friend additional copies for Alex.

Although this arrangement is not perfect (nothing is), it gives Alex the best chance to stay on top of things and not get so far behind that he is lost and frustrated when he returns to class. Although the teacher probably won't mind quickly going over the makeup work with the friend at the end of the period, she cannot be expected to *remember* to send assignment lists, study sheets, makeup sheets, and personal notes to the office each day that your son is absent. If Alex does not have any friends who can help out and the teacher is unwilling or unable to appoint a child to take on the responsibility, you might have to arrange with each teacher to pick up the assignments and paperwork; alternatively, it might be possible for the teacher to e-mail the assignments to Alex.

I know such arrangements sound difficult and complicated, but your diligence will make the difference in whether Alex feels that he is part of the classes when he is there. If he keeps up with the work when he's at home, he'll know what's going on, be able to participate in class, and he won't be overwhelmed by the stress that usually comes with being absent.

My daughter, Laura, has an individualized education plan (IEP). In addition to her chronic headaches, she has ADHD (attention-deficit/hyperactivity disorder) of the primarily inattentive type and needs to sit near the front of the room, take extra time on tests, and fill out an assignment sheet each day. All this information is in her IEP, which was given to each of Laura's teachers (she is in seventh grade). Should I sit back at the beginning of the school year and see how things go before I meet with her teachers, or should I meet with her teachers at the very beginning of the year, before they have gotten to know her? Laura is a very sweet girl who causes no problems in class.

[C. Freeman:] In thinking about this question, it is important to note that Laura has an IEP, not just a "problem with school." She has been officially tested, and it has been determined that for Laura to succeed in school, she *needs* certain accommodations or modifications in her learning environment. It is because she *needs* help that the school district is willing, and legally obligated, to provide it.

Students with IEPs usually have serious *academic*, or *learning*, problems that prevent them from meeting the standards of the class. Parents of a student with physical, emotional, or learning disabilities can submit a "request for special education assessment." An evaluation is then made to see whether the student qualifies for special accommodations and modifications under an IEP.

For the students who do not have IEPs, I make it a rule at the beginning of each semester not to look in any "cum cards" (cumulative records of grades, standardized tests, teacher's comments) for at least a month. I want each student to have a fresh start, and I don't want to pre-judge anyone on the basis of past performance or behavior.

Laura, however, is in a different situation. Because she has a current IEP, there is no reason (except wishful thinking) to think that her problems are going to go away. It is reasonable to expect that her problems will be helped only if the recommendations in the IEP are followed. It is important that you speak with each of Laura's teachers at the beginning of each semester. A child with ADHD of any type has trouble focusing and staying on task. A child with ADHD of the primarily inattentive type daydreams quietly—weeks could go by before the teacher notices that there's a problem. (This is very different from a child with ADHD of the primarily hyperactive type—this child rarely goes unnoticed!)

You might reasonably say that Laura's teachers were given copies of her IEP, and they know what adaptations and modifications need to be made. Why do you need to "bug" them by coming in and telling them exactly what is in the IEP? The reason is simple—with all the paperwork teachers receive (seventh-grade teachers usually have five or six classes plus a homeroom), they usually look over the IEPs quickly and then put them in a drawer. A good teacher makes a note in the roll book that the student has an IEP. You want more than that. Each time the teacher looks at your daughter, the teacher should be thinking, *That's Laura, who has problems focusing.* When the teacher sees Laura staring out the window, you don't want the teacher to lose patience and to embarrass Laura by reprimanding her to turn around and pay attention. The teacher needs to bear in mind that Laura has an IEP and go quietly over to Laura to remind her to focus on what is being taught in class. You want the teacher to remember *Laura has a problem*, rather than to think, *Laura is a problem.* You also want the teacher to know from the beginning that you, Laura's parent, are concerned, supportive, and involved.

After the initial meeting, it is important to check with each teacher at least once a month to make sure that everything is going well and that

Laura's needs are being met. Most good teachers appreciate the reminder. The bad ones need reminding even if they don't like it! Don't expect Laura to tell you that she is not paying attention, not doing her work, or getting into trouble. Children tend to think that if they say nothing, the problem will go away. Unfortunately, it just escalates until the teacher finally makes a call, by which time the problem is much more difficult to fix.

My 12-year-old son, Victor, goes to a school where hats are not allowed. He has to wear a hat in school because he had a scalp condition that left his head very sensitive. He began having headaches and learned that wearing a hat helped reduce his headaches. His doctor also thought wearing a hat during the day was a good idea, because Victor was missing a lot of school before he started wearing the hat. Besides informing the school of his condition and need, what can I do to help my child cope with children making fun of him and adults confronting him about not following the school rules?

[C. Freeman:] Victor's attitude toward wearing his hat, to a large extent, will determine whether he is picked on or accepted by his peers. The first thing to do is buy Victor a "cool" hat rather than a "dorky" one. (Also make sure that the hat is not of a type associated with any gangs!) You want this hat to be either the envy of the other students (they wish they could wear a hat like that to school) or unremarkable. Next, figure out with Victor a simple explanation that he is going to give the other students when they ask him why he is allowed to wear a hat in school. It can be as simple as "I have a scalp problem and need to wear a hat" or "It's a medical thing."

At this point, if Victor still comes home complaining that the students are making fun of him, you have to look deeper into the problem. The problem might no longer be the hat—it might be either Victor's attitude or explanation about the hat (e.g., he could be covering up embarrassment by telling classmates he gets to wear the hat because he is "special") or a peer problem that has nothing to do with the hat.

Dealing with the adults at school can pose another problem for Victor. He should have no problem with his teachers, the school nurse, and anyone else who knows him personally. A "confidential health card" explaining his condition will be passed around to all of his teachers, and each teacher will be required to initial the card. The problem comes up when an adult he doesn't know approaches him and asks him why he is wearing a hat in school. Any adult in authority on campus needs to know only that Victor has permission to wear the hat. Therefore, Victor needs to get a note from the school nurse or principal stating that it is okay for him to wear a hat. He should keep this note with him at all times (as he would money) and hand it to any adult who questions him. To his friends, it will look like he has a "get out of jail free" pass, and the adults will leave him alone as soon as they see the note.

Patty, my 10-year-old daughter, suffers from fibromyalgia. She has a low energy level, is sometimes dizzy, and has frequent headaches. What should she do in school when she feels dizzy, has a headache, or gets tired? She is afraid her teacher won't believe her.

[C. Freeman:] You are dealing with two main issues here. First, the school must accommodate Patty when dizziness or pain occurs during the school day. Second, Patty must be motivated to go to school and work despite feeling tired a large part of the time and sometimes dizzy. To secure the accommodations Patty needs, you will have to speak with the school nurse and Patty's teacher. The nurse needs a letter from Patty's doctor documenting that Patty has a legitimate medical diagnosis. (Fibromyalgia is a legitimate medical diagnosis of a type of pain disorder.) The teacher has to understand that Patty is not making up the dizziness and headaches; she is not faking it. Perhaps, when she is dizzy, another child can accompany her to the nurse's office. If the teacher objects to Patty leaving the room so often, you have options.

You can request that Patty be evaluated to determine whether she qualifies for school accommodations under Section 504 of IDEA. This would force the teacher to make the appropriate accommodations for Patty. Better yet, you can go to the principal or director of the school to request another teacher for Patty. (This does not preclude you from requesting a 504 plan to ensure that in the future Patty's special needs are met.) She does not need tutoring from a resource teacher; this would only cause her to miss more classroom time. She only needs to be allowed to leave class when she is suffering. This arrangement will allow Patty the benefits of staying in school rather than missing school.

Arrangements also need to be made with the school nurse as to what will happen when Patty goes to the nurse's office. In addition to the doctor's letter, it might be helpful if the nurse speaks to Patty's doctor. Instead of sending Patty home, the nurse might be able to provide a quiet setting where Patty can use relaxation techniques to ease her pain. If certain medications are appropriate, you should provide the nurse with these medications and with instructions signed by Patty's doctor stating when, what, and how much medication should be given. Although with a doctor's order Patty legally may carry medication, because of her young age and the problem with illegal drugs—and because some schools have rules prohibiting this—it is preferable that the medication be kept in the nurse's office.

CONCLUSION—AND THE GOLDEN RULES OF CHRONIC PAIN

My goal in writing this book has been to give you the tools to be informed parents and to trust your instincts when it comes to your child. I hope I have accomplished this. After this chapter, there is a list of pediatric pain programs around the country that you may consult for further advice, as well as Web sites and books on pain and related subjects that I hope will be of further help to you.

The path to wellness is not always linear. There can and will be many bends in the road, but the journey is often filled with wonderful surprises that will strengthen your family, make you a better parent, and leave you with a happier and healthier child.

I am in complete awe of the parents and children I see who struggle with chronic pain on a daily basis. I am constantly amazed at their strength, resourcefulness, and sense of humor even in the face of unimaginable pain and frustration. On those days when I am overwhelmed with work and am questioning myself, I think of them and I am reminded why I do what I do.

I want to leave you with a list we have developed in our pain program; we call it the "Golden Rules of Chronic Pain." Copy this list and post it on the refrigerator, or wherever you will see it every day.

Golden Rules of Chronic Pain

All Pain Is Real

Pain is caused by a complex interaction between the brain and the rest of the body. If the body has been in pain for a long time, the nervous system can continue sending pain signals even if there is no longer any tissue damage. This is why many patients are told "there is nothing medically wrong," or "it must be psychological." In fact, pain is neurological.

Improvement Is First Measured by Increased Functioning

Your child is improving when you see an improvement in her day-to-day functioning. For most patients, the pain goes away *after* the child is functioning normally.

Don't Ask Your Child If She Is in Pain

Pain is worse when you are paying attention to it and better if you are distracted from it. If you ask your child if she is in pain, she will scan her body looking for the pain and find it. If she happens to be distracted from the pain at that moment, we want that moment to be continued. It is perfectly fine for her to complain to you if she feels pain, however.

Exercise Is Good for Sleep and for Chronic Pain

Nonimpact aerobic exercise is good for everyone, especially for your child. Moderate exercise not only helps to improve the immune system but also improves the pain-relief response from the brain and puts the body and brain in better overall health.

Sleep Is Good

Impaired sleep is directly related to chronic pain. It is helpful to have a regular routine to regulate sleep. It is recommended that your child go to bed at the same time each night, get up at the same time each day, and use the bed only for sleeping (not for doing homework or watching TV).

Reduce Anxiety

Anxiety does not cause pain. However, it makes all types of pain worse (even cancer pain). If your child has anxiety or worries, it is extremely important to obtain appropriate treatment for three reasons: (1) reducing anxiety makes pain better; (2) reducing anxiety speeds recovery from many medical disorders; (3) reducing anxiety makes the rest of your child's life better.

A Long-Term Problem Requires a Long-Term Solution

Quick solutions do not work for chronic pain problems. Children who do best over time make slow and steady progress in functioning first. If your child has been in pain for a long time, it will likely take a similar amount of time for the pain to resolve.

Glossary of Useful Pain Terminology

arthralgia: Arthritis-like pain that occurs in joints but without any noticeable inflammation. For example, you can have arthralgias during the flu, even though there is no actual inflammation of the joints.

arthritis: An inflammatory condition of the joints associated with joint pain, such as juvenile rheumatoid arthritis (JRA).

Asperger's syndrome: A developmental condition characterized by social interaction problems, difficulty reading nonverbal cues, difficulties with transitions or changes, preference for routine and rituals, clumsiness, unusual preoccupations, and normal language development. (*See* autism spectrum disorder.)

autism spectrum disorder (ASD): A developmental condition characterized by a delay in the acquisition of language, repetitive mannerisms and interests, a strong preference for routines and rituals, lack of imaginative play, severe social difficulties, poor eye contact, and a lack of interest in others.

autonomic nervous system (ANS): The portion of the nervous system that regulates involuntary body functions, including those of the heart and intestine. Controls blood flow, digestion, and temperature regulation.

clinical trials: Carefully planned and monitored experiments to test a new drug or treatment. Unfortunately, there are few clinical trials involving children. Some of the pediatric pain programs in Appendix B can be contacted to see if they have clinical pain trials for children. The National Institutes of Health Web site, www.nih.org, also has a list of pediatric clinical trials.

cognitive-behavioral therapy (CBT): A treatment strategy used to teach a child how to identify things and situations that stress him, and how to control anxiety associated with those stressors. It strives to replace anxiety-producing thoughts and behaviors with new ones until the stressors no longer make the child anxious.

central nervous system (CNS): The brain, spinal cord, and spinal nerves. The CNS serves as the main processing center for the whole nervous system, and thus controls all the workings of the body.

complementary and alternative medicine (CAM): Approaches to medical treatment that are outside of mainstream medical training (e.g., acupuncture, meditation, aromatherapy, Chinese medicine, dance therapy, music therapy, massage, herbal medicine, therapeutic touch, yoga, chiropractic, naturopathy, and homeopathy).

complex regional pain syndrome (CRPS): A neuropathic pain condition (formerly called reflex sympathetic dystrophy, or RSD) in which sensory nerves to a certain regional part of the body get turned on and that area becomes supersensitive, so that even light touch can be painful.

computed tomography scan (CT scan): An x-ray technique that uses a computer to construct cross-sectional images of the body.

electrical stimulation: Application of currents to induce pain relief, such as transcutaneous electrical nerve stimulation (TENS).

endorphins: Naturally occurring molecules made up of amino acids. Endorphins attach to special receptors in the brain and spinal cord to stop pain messages. These are the same receptors that respond to morphine.

enkephalins: (Pronounced *en-KEF-uh-lins.*) Naturally occurring molecules in the brain. Enkephalins attach to special receptors in your brain and spinal cord to stop pain messages. They also affect other functions within the brain and nervous system.

fibromyalgia: A disorder characterized by fatigue, stiffness, joint tenderness, and widespread muscle pain. Juvenile fibromyalgia is different from adult-onset fibromyalgia, in that children can outgrow the former.

functional abdominal pain (FAP): A functional gastrointestinal (GI) condition with belly pain (no other GI symptoms) caused by disordered brain–gut nerve signaling.

functional dyspepsia: A painful functional GI condition in the midupper abdomen (ulcer location but no ulcer) caused by disordered brain–gut nerve signaling.

functional pain: Pain that is not derived from infection, inflammation, injury, or structural damage. It is related to the abnormal and disordered function of nerve signals that send increased pain messages to the brain.

gastroenterology: The branch of medicine dealing with the study of disorders affecting the stomach, intestines, and associated organs.

gastrointestinal (GI): Related to the stomach and intestines.

general anesthesia: A state of unconsciousness induced by a medication that eliminates pain perception.

headaches: Pain in the head. Tension (muscular) headaches can feel like pressure or throbbing; migraines are often throbbing and can be associated with nausea and visual disturbances.

individualized education plan (IEP): Parents of a student with physical, emotional, or learning disabilities can submit a "request for special education assessment." An evaluation is then made to see whether the student qualifies for special accommodations and modifications under an IEP. Students with IEPs usually have serious academic or learning problems that prevent them from meeting the standards of the class.

inflammatory bowel disease (IBD): Intestinal disease related to intestinal inflammation and associated with diarrhea, bleeding, cramping, obstruction (a blockage of the intestine), malabsorption (failure of the intestines to absorb minerals and nutrients), and weight loss or poor weight gain (e.g., ulcerative colitis, Crohn's disease).

irritable bowel syndrome (IBS): A functional GI condition with belly pain and nausea, vomiting, bloating, diarrhea, or constipation, and caused by disordered brain–gut nerve signaling.

juvenile rheumatoid arthritis (JRA): An autoimmune condition in children that involves primarily pain and inflammation in the joints. There are a number of differences between JRA and adult rheumatoid arthritis.

limbic center: The portion of the brain that produces emotions. This is the core of the "emotional brain."

magnetic resonance imaging (MRI): A technique used in a medical setting to produce high-quality images of the inside of the body.

musculoskeletal: relating to or involving the muscles and the skeleton.

myofascial pain: Pain and tenderness in the muscles and adjacent fibrous tissues (fascia) with sensitive areas known as trigger or tender points located within the body's muscles.

narcotic: (*See* opioid.)

nervous system: Generally refers to three body systems: (1) the central nervous system (CNS), which is the brain and spinal cord; (2) the peripheral nervous system, which is the cervical, thoracic, lumbar, and sacral nerve trunks leading away from the spine to the limbs; and (3) the autonomic nervous system (ANS), which has cell bodies alongside the spinal cord with nerves that travel back and forth to internal organs, the body's periphery, and to a central area in the brainstem.

neuromodule: Pain circuits within the cortical (conscious) areas of the brain.

neurotransmitters: The naturally occurring chemicals in human beings and animals that relay electrical messages among the nerve cells. The three neurotransmitters we are most familiar with are serotonin, norepinephrine, and dopamine.

nociceptors: (Pronounced *no-sih-SEP-turs*.) Special small nerve fibers that carry pain or negative sensory messages.

neuropsychology: The study of brain/behavior relationships. Neuropsychologists have extensive training in the anatomy, physiology, and pathology of the nervous system and in how these systems affect thinking and emotions. Clinical child neuropsychologists evaluate cognitive (thinking and performing) function in children and make recommendations for treatment to improve function on the basis of the test results and their observations of the child. Cognitive testing can be helpful for children with suspected learning disabilities or uneven IQ.

opioid: Prescription medication that relieves pain by binding to specialized receptors in the brain and spinal cord. Some are derived from opium; others are synthetic (same as narcotics.) (For natural opioids, *see* enkephalins.)

pain: An unpleasant sensory and emotional experience associated with actual or potential tissue damage or described in terms of such damage (definition from the International Association for the Study of Pain).

pain-associated disability syndrome (PADS): A condition in which a child with chronic pain functions less and less well over time (e.g., not attending school, sleeping poorly, not playing with friends, not physically active).

parasympathetic nervous system (PNS): The part of the autonomic nervous system (ANS) responsible for restorative functions such as digestion.

patient-controlled analgesia (PCA): A computerized system that allows a patient to control the amount of pain medicine he receives.

The patient pushes a button and a machine delivers a preset dose of pain medicine into the bloodstream through a vein.

peripheral nerves: Nerves that run from your spinal cord to all other parts of your body. They transmit messages from the spinal cord and the brain to and from other parts of your body, and send sensory signals back to the spinal cord and brain.

perseverative: Tending to stay with one thing and not let go. The word is often used to describe children with pervasive developmental disorders (PDD) such as autism.

pervasive developmental disorder (PDD): A neurological condition associated with a broad range of cognitive and behavioral abnormalities, but always including a deficit in social perception and interaction (problems with emotional intelligence).

phantom pain: Pain or discomfort after amputation that feels as if it comes from the missing limb or organ.

physical therapy (PT): A treatment in which muscles and ligaments are stretched, balanced, and strengthened.

placebo: A supposedly inert/inactive substance (e.g., sugar pill, saline injection), psychological, or behavioral treatment that is used in clinical studies as control factors to help determine the efficacy of active treatments. However, more recent research has shown that placebos can also have active effects.

recurrent pain: Pain that occurs or appears again or repeatedly.

reflex sympathetic dystrophy (RSD): (*See* complex regional pain syndrome.)

rehabilitation: A treatment aimed at restoring function.

relaxation: A condition in which the muscles are loose; stress hormones are low; heart rate, breathing rate, and blood pressure are normal or low; and the body feels warm and comfortable. Relaxation techniques are strategies used to attain a state of relaxation.

selective serotonin reuptake inhibitors (SSRIs): Medications used to relieve depression and anxiety. May work by increasing the availability of a brain chemical that helps to regulate mood (serotonin).

side effects: Unwanted changes produced by medication or other treatment, ranging from minor and temporary, such as dry mouth, to more serious, such as gastrointestinal (GI) bleeding.

sign: An objective finding such as *what* a doctor notices in a patient. Examples are a heart murmur, an enlarged liver, or a rash. (*See* symptom.)

spinal cord: A cordlike bundle of nerves that extends from the base of the brain to the small of the back. The dorsal part (outer half toward the back) of the spinal cord carries the nerve fibers that relay pain messages to the brain.

sympathetic nervous system (SNS): The part of the autonomic nervous system (ANS) responsible for fight-or-flight reactions (e.g., speeding up of heartbeat and breathing, increased sweating).

symptom: What your child tells you he is feeling, such as pain, nausea, or bloating. (*See* sign.)

tricyclic antidepressants: A group of drugs used in high doses to relieve symptoms of depression and in low doses to relieve certain types of pain (e.g., irritable bowel syndrome, neuropathic pain).

trigger point: A hypersensitive area or site in muscle or connective tissue at which touch or pressure will elicit pain.

{ APPENDIX B }

Pediatric Pain and Gastrointestinal Pain Programs

GENERAL PAIN PROGRAMS

United States

UCLA Pediatric Pain Program, UCLA Mattel Children's Hospital, David Geffen School of Medicine at UCLA; 10833 Le Conte Ave. #22-464 MDCC, **Los Angeles, CA** 90095; Lonnie Zeltzer, M.D.; phone: 310-825-0731; fax: 310-794-2104; lzeltzer@mednet.ucla.edu; www.healthcare.ucla.edu/pedspain

The Children's Hospital, Chronic Pain Clinic, Department of Anesthesiology; B090, 1056 East 19th Ave., **Denver, CO** 80218; Glenn Merritt, M.D., and Roxie Foster, Ph.D., R.N.; phone: 303-861-6226; fax: 303-837-2899; wahlstrom.julie@tchden.org

The Children's Hospital & Regional Medical Center, Children's Pain
Management Program; 4800 Sandpoint Way NE, **Seattle, WA** 98105-
0371; Corrie Anderson, M.D.; phone: 206-528-2704; fax: 206-527-3935;
www.seattlechildrens.org

Children's Hospital Los Angeles, Comfort and Pain Management
Program; 4650 Sunset Blvd., MS #3, **Los Angeles, CA** 90027-6062;
Michael H. Joseph, M.D.; phone: 323-660-2450, x6347; fax: 323-660-8983

Children's Hospitals and Clinics, Integrative Medicine Program, 2525
Chicago Ave. South, **Minneapolis, MN** 55404; Timothy Culbert, M.D.;
phone: 612-813-7888; fax: 612-813-7199; timothy.culbert@childrenshc.org;
www.childrensintegrativemed.org

Children's Hospital, Pain Treatment Service, 300 Longwood Ave.,
Boston, MA 02115; Charles B. Berde, M.D., Ph.D.; phone: 617-355-6995;
fax: 617-730-0199; www.childrenshospital.org

Children's Memorial Hospital, Northwestern University, Feinberg
School of Medicine, 2300 Children's Plaza, **Chicago, IL** 60614;
Santhanam Suresh, M.D., FAAP; Patrick Birmingham, M.D., FAAP;
phone: 773-880-4006; fax: 773-880-3331; www.childrensmemorial.org

Cincinnati Children's Hospital Medical Center, Division of Pain
Management, 3333 Burnet Ave., **Cincinnati, OH** 45229-3039;
Kenneth R. Goldschneider, M.D., FAAP; phone: 513-636-7768;
fax: 513-636-2920; kenneth.goldschneider@cchmc.org;
www.cincinnatichildrens.org/svc/prog/pain-clinic/default.htm

Pediatric Pain Management Program, Children's Hospital of New York–Presbyterian, BH-440N; 622 West 168th St.; **New York, NY** 10032; William Schechter, M.D.; phone: 212-305-7114; ws5@columbia.edu

Comprehensive Chronic Pain Management Center for Children and Adolescents, Kennedy Krieger Institute, Johns Hopkins University School of Medicine, 707 North Broadway, **Baltimore, MD** 21205; Jim Christensen, M.D.; phone: 443-923-9414; fax: 443-923-9405; luttrell@kennedykrieger.org

The David Center for Children's Pain and Palliative Care, Hackensack University Medical Center, 30 Prospect Ave., **Hackensack, NJ** 07601; Gary A. Walco, Ph.D.; phone: 201-996-DAVE (-3283); fax: 201-487-7340; gwalco@humed.com; www.thechildrenshospitalhumc.net/s199/index.asp?LOB=199

Doernbecher/OHSU, Pediatric Pain Management Center, 3181 SW Sam Jackson Park Rd., UHS 2, **Portland, OR** 97239-3098; Jeffrey L. Koh, M.D., MBA; phone: 503-418-5188; fax: 503-418-5340

Jane B. Pettit Pain and Palliative Care Center, Medical College of Wisconsin, 9000 West Wisconsin Ave. MS 792, **Milwaukee, WI** 53226; Steven J. Weisman, M.D.; phone: 414-266-2775; fax: 414-266-1761

Lucile Packard Children's Hospital at Stanford, 725 Welch Rd., **Palo Alto, CA** 94304; Elliot Krane, M.D.; phone: 650-724-5338; fax: 650-725-5344; krane@stanford.edu; pedsanesthesia.stanford.edu

Mayo Clinic, Rochester Pediatric Pain Management Clinic, Eisenberg
8G, 200 First St.; SW; **Rochester, MN** 55905; Robert T. Wilder, M.D.,
Ph.D.; phone: 507-266-9240; fax: 507-266-7732; wilder.robert@mayo.edu

The Pain Management Program; Children's Hospital of Philadelphia,
University of Pennsylvania, 34th and Civic Center Blvd.; **Philadelphia,
PA** 19104; John B. Rose, M.D.; phone: 215-590-1409; fax: 215-590-1415;
rose@email.chop.edu

Pediatric Pain and Palliative Care, Methodist Children's Hospital, 7700
Floyd Curl Drive, **San Antonio, TX 78229**; Amanda Dove, M.D.;
Cindy Wall, MSN, R.N., CNS; phone: 210-575-7497; cindy.wall@
mhshealth.com; www.sahealth.com

Pain Relief Program, Connecticut Children's Medical Center, 282
Washington St., **Hartford, CT** 06106; Neil Schechter, MD;
860-545-9997; Fax: 860-545-8661

Pediatric Pain Evaluation Clinic and Pediatric Rheumatology Program,
Duke University Medical Center 3212; **Durham, NC** 27710;
Laura Schanberg, M.D.; phone: 919-684-6575; fax: 919-684-6616;
www.dukehealth.org

Pediatric Rheumatology Program, University of Kansas Medical Center,
Department of Pediatrics, 3901 Rainbow Blvd., **Kansas City, KS**
66160-7330; Carol Lindsley, M.D.; Michael Rapoff, Ph.D.;
phone: 913-588-588-6325; fax: 913-588-9319; clindsley@kumc.edu;
mrapoff@kumc.edu; www2.kumc.edu/kids

St. Mary's Health Care System for Children, Pain Management Program, 29-01 2216th St., **Bayside, NY** 11360; Alice Olwell, R.N.; phone: 718-281-8749; fax: 718-279-2141; aolwell@stmaryskids.org; www.stmaryskids.org

The Jason Program, 13 Industrial Park Rd., **Saco, ME** 04072; Gary Allegretta, M.D., and Kate Swain Eastman, Psy.D., LCSW; phone: 207-294-8255; fax 207-294-8257; programdirector@jasonprogram.org; www.jasonprogram.org

Trinity KidsCare Hospice, 2601 Airport Drive, suite 230, **Torrance, CA** 90505; Gayle C. Kirma, LCSW; phone: 310-530-3800; fax: 310-534-5095; gayle.kirma@providence.org; www.trinitycarehospice.org

Pediatric Advanced Care Team, Children's Hospital Boston and Dana-Farber Cancer Institute, 44 Binney St., **Boston, MA** 02115; Joanne Wolfe, M.D., MPH; phone: 617-632-5042; fax: 617-632-2270; janet.duncan@childrens.harvard.edu

University of New Mexico Pediatric Pain Clinic, 1213 University Blvd. NE, **Albuquerque, NM** 87102; Eileen D. Yager, M.D.; phone: 505-925-4994; fax: 505-925-4919; eyager@salud.unm.edu

Yale New Haven Children's Hospital, Pediatric Pain Management Services, 333 Cedar St. TMP-3, P.O. Box 208051; **New Haven, CT** 06520-8051; Brenda C. McClain, M.D., DABPM; phone: 203-785-2802; fax: 203-688-7979 or 203-688-6664; brenda.mcclain@yale.edu; www.ynhh.org/ynhch/ynhch.html

Canada

Complex Pain Service, Integrated Pain Service, BC Children's Hospital, 4480 Oak St., **Vancouver, British Columbia** V6H 3N4, **Canada**; phone: 604-875-2000, local 5108; Tim F. Oberlander, M.D., FRCPC; toberlander@cw.bc.ca

Chronic Pain Program, Hospital for Sick Children, 555 University Ave.; **Toronto, Ontario, Canada,** M5G 1X8; Stephen C. Brown, M.D.; phone: 416-813-7445; fax: 416-813-7543; stephen.brown@sickkids.ca

IWK Health Centre Pediatric Pain Clinic, Dalhousie University, 5850 University Ave., **Halifax, Nova Scotia** B3J 3G9, **Canada**; G. Allen Finley, M.D., FRCPC, FAAP; phone: 902.470.8769; fax: 902-470-7911; paula.forgeron@iwk.nshealth.ca; www.pediatric-pain.ca

The Montreal Children's Hospital of the McGill University Health Centre, Chronic Pain Management Centre, 2300 rue Tupper, C-1117, **Montréal, Québec** H3H 1P3, **Canada**; Joëlle Desparmet, M.D.; info@thechildren.com

International

Children's Pain Management Service, Royal Children's Hospital (Melbourne), Flemington Rd., **Parkville, Victoria** 3052, **Australia**; George Chalkiadis, M.D.; phone: 61-3-9345-5233; fax: 61-3-9345-6003; stephanie.dowden@rch.org.au; www.rch.org.au/anaes/index.cfm? doc_id=778

Chronic Pain Service, Sydney Children's Hospital, High St., Randwick, 2031, **New South Wales, Australia**; Matthew Crawford, M.D.; phone: 61-2-9382-1625; fax: 61-2-9382-1896; m.mcinerney@unsw.edu.au

Pain and Palliative Care Service, Children's Hospital at Westmead, Locked Bag 4001, **Westmead, Sydney** NSW 2145, **Australia**; John J. Collins, M.B. B.S.; Ph.D., FRACP; phone: 61-2-9845-0000; fax: 61-2-9845-3421; michaelc@chw.edu.au; www.chw.edu.au

Starship Hospital Pain Clinic, Starship Hospital, Park Rd., Grafton, **Auckland, New Zealand**; Dr. Malcolm Futter-FRCA, FANZCA; phone: 09-307-4949; fax: 09-375-4368; malcolmf@adhb.govt.nz

Institute of Pediatric Pain Therapy and Palliative Care (Institut für Kinderschmerztherapie und Pädiatrische Palliativmedizin), Children's Hospital and Clinic (Vestische Kinderklinik), University of Witten (Herdecke); Friedrich Steiner, M.D.; Str. 5, 45711 **Datteln, Germany**; Boris Zernikow, M.D.; phone: 49-2363-975-180; fax: 49-2363-64211; boris.zernikow@t-online.de; www.schmerzen-bei-kindern.de

Pain Management Unit, Royal National Hospital for Rheumatic Diseases, NHS Trust, Upper Borough Walls, **Bath**, BA1 1RL; **United Kingdom**; Dr. Jacqui Clinch (Medical Director), M.D.; Dr. Hannah Connell; phone: 44-0-1225-473427; fax: 44-0-1225-421202; pain@bath.ac.uk; www.bath.ac.uk/psychology/pmu

Pain Therapy, Pediatric Department, University of Padova, Italy, Via Giustiniani 3, **Padova, Italy**; Dr. Franca Benini; phone: 39-049-8211899; fax: 39-049-8213509; benini@pediatria.unipd.it; http://www.pediatria.unipd.it

Queen Paola Children's Hospital, Lindendreef 1-2020 **Antwerp, Belgium**, Gigi Veereman-Wauters M.D., Ph.D.; phone: 0032-2802200/0032 -2802291; fax: 0032-2802133

PEDIATRIC GASTROENTEROLOGY PROGRAMS SPECIALIZING IN FUNCTIONAL BOWEL DISORDERS

United States

Center for Functional Gastrointestinal and Motility Disorders; Goryeb Children's Hospital; 100 Madison Ave., Box 82; **Morristown, NJ** 07962; Nader N. Youssef, M.D., MBA; phone: 973-971-5676; fax: 973-290-7365; nader.youssef@ahsys.org

Children's Hospital, 747 52nd St.; **Oakland, CA** 94609; Elizabeth Gleghorn, M.D.; phone: 570-428-3058; fax: 570-450-5813

Children's Digestive Health Center, Children's Hospital of New York–Presbyterian, 3959 Broadway, **New York, NY** 10032; Joseph (Yosi) Levy, M.D.; phone: 212-305-5693; fax: 212-305-7124; j1588@columbia.edu

Children's Center for Digestive Health Care, 993-D Johnson Ferry Rd., #440, **Atlanta, GA** 30342; phone: 404-257-0799; fax: 404-256-5475; www.ccdhc.org

Children's Memorial Hospital, Cyclic Vomiting Program, 2300 Children's Plaza, #57, **Chicago, IL** 60614-3394; B.U.K. Li, M.D.; phone: 773-880-4496; fax: 773-880-4036; cvscenter@childrensmemorial.org

Digestive Diseases and Nutrition, Connecticut Children's Medical Center, 282 Washington St.; **Hartford, CT** 06106; Jeffrey Hyams, M.D.; phone: 860-545-9560

Division of Pediatric Gastroenterology, Ronald McDonald Children's Hospital, Loyola University Medical Center, 2160 South First Ave., **Maywood, IL** 60153; James H. Berman, M.D.; phone: 708-327-9073; fax: 708-327-9160; JBerma@lumc.edu

Pediatric Gastroenterology, 545 Valley View Drive; **Moline, IL** 62165; Mohammad Yaseen, M.D.; phone: 309-762-5560; fax: 309-762-7351; mya2024231@aol.com

Division of Pediatric Gastroenterology and Nutrition, Stony Brook University Hospital, **Stony Brook, NY** 11794; Anupama Chawla, M.D.; phone: 631-444-8115; fax: 631-444-6045

Division of Pediatric Gastroenterology, Kansas University Children's Center, 3901 Rainbow Blvd., **Kansas City, KS** 66160; Paul E Hyman, M.D.; phone: 913-588-6819; phyman@kumc.edu

Division of Pediatric Gastroenterology, Kennedy Krieger Institute, 707 North Broadway, **Baltimore, MD** 21205; Anil Darbari, M.D.; phone: 443-923-9440; fax: 443-923-2645; www.kennedykrieger.org

Division of Pediatric Gastroenterology, Rush Children's Hospital, 1653 West Congress Parkway, **Chicago, IL** 60612; Richard H. Sandler, M.D.; phone: 312-942-2889; fax: 312-563-2131; www.rush.edu/rumc/page-R12224.html

Division of Pediatric Gastroenterology, University of Nevada School of Medicine, 3196 Maryland Pkwy, #309; **Las Vegas, NV** 89109; Howard Baron, M.D.; phone: 702-791-0477; fax: 702-791-6831

Pediatric Gastroenterology, Hepatology, and Nutrition, Vanderbilt University Medical Center, **Nashville, TN** 37232; D. Brent Polk, M.D.; phone: 615-322-7449; www.vanderbiltchildrens.com

Canada

Hôpital Sainte-Justine, 3175 Côte Sainte-Catherine, **Montréal, Québec** H3T 1C5, **Canada**; Andrée Rasquin, M.D.; phone: 514-345-4626; fax: 514-345-4999; a.rasquin@umontreal.ca

McMaster Children's Hospital; 1200 Main St. West; **Hamilton, Ontario**, L8N 3Z5, **Canada**; Robert Issenman, M.D.; phone: 905-521-2655

International

Royal Children's Hospital and District Health Service, Herston Rd., **Herston, Brisbane**, QLD 4029, **Australia**; Looi Ee, M.D.; phone: 61-7-3636-7887; fax: 61-7-3636-3472; www.rchf.org.au/

Queen Paola Children's Hospital, Lindendreef 1-2020, **Antwerp, Belgium**; Professor Micheline Van Caillie-Bertrand; phone: 0032-2802200/0032-2802291; fax: 0032-2802133

{ APPENDIX C }

Selected Readings

BOOKS

Attwood, Tony, and Lorna Wing: *Asperger's Syndrome: A Guide for Parents and Professionals*. London: Jessica Kingsley Publishers, 1998.

Bourne, Edmund J.: *Anxiety and Phobia Workbook*, 3rd ed. Oakland, CA: New Harbinger Press, 2000.

Cheyette, Sarah: *Mommy, My Head Hurts: A Doctor's Guide to Your Child's Headache*. New York: Newmarket Press, 2002.

Cohen, Shirley: *Targeting Autism: What We Know, Don't Know, and Can Do to Help Young Children with Autism and Related Disorders*. Berkeley, CA: University of California Press, 2002 (updated).

Diamond, Seymour, with Amy Diamond: *Headache and Your Child: The Complete Guide to Understanding and Treating Migraine and Other Headaches in Children and Adolescents*. New York: Fireside, 2001.

Ferber, Richard: *Solve Your Child's Sleep Problems*. New York: Fireside, 1996.

Grandin, Temple: *Emergence: Labeled Autistic*. New York: Warner Books, 1996.

Grandin, Temple: *Thinking in Pictures: And Other Reports from My Life with Autism*. New York: Vintage, 1996.

Greene, Ross W.: *The Explosive Child: A New Approach for Understanding and Parenting Easily Frustrated, Chronically Inflexible Children*, 2nd ed. New York: HarperCollins, 2001.

Hallowell, M.D., Edward M.: *Worry: Controlling It and Using It Wisely*. New York: Ballantine, 1998.

Hartzell, Mary, and Dan Siegel: *Parenting from the Inside Out: How a Deeper Self-Understanding Can Help You Raise Children Who Thrive*. New York: J.P. Tarcher, 2003.

Iyengar, B.K.S.: *The Path to Holistic Health*. New York: Dorling Kindersley, 2001.

Jackson, Luke, and Tony Attwood: *Freaks, Geeks and Asperger Syndrome: A User Guide to Adolescence*. London: Jessica Kingsley, 2002.

Kabat-Zinn, Jon, and Myla Kabat-Zinn: *Everyday Blessings: The Inner Work of Mindful Parenting*, 2nd ed. New York: Hyperion, 1998.

Krane, Elliot: *Make the Pain Go Away, Mommy!: A Doctor's Revolutionary Approach to End Your Child's Chronic Pain and Suffering*. New York: Fireside Books, in press.

Kranowitz, Carol Stock, and Larry B. Silver: *The Out-of-Sync Child: Recognizing and Coping with Sensory Integration Dysfunction*. New York: Perigee, 1998.

Levy, Joseph: *My Tummy Hurts: A Complete Guide to Understanding and Treating Your Child's Stomachaches*. New York: Fireside, 2004.

Maurice, Catherine: *Let Me Hear Your Voice: A Family's Triumph Over Autism*. New York: Ballantine, 1994.

Olness, Karen, and Dan P. Kohen: *Hypnosis and Hypnotherapy with Children*, 3rd ed. New York: Guilford Press, 1996.

Schatz, Mary Pullig: *Back Care Basics*. Berkeley, CA: Rodmell Press, 1992.

Seroussi, Karen: *Unraveling the Mystery of Autism and Pervasive Developmental Disorder: A Mother's Story of Research and Recovery*. New York: Broadway, 2002.

Shaw, William: *Biological Treatments for Autism and PDD*, 2nd ed. Overland Park, KS: Great Plains Laboratory, 2001.

Sparrowe, Linda, and Patricia Walden: *The Woman's Book of Yoga and Health*. Boston: Shambhala Publications, 2002.

Zeltzer, Paul: *Brain Tumors: Finding the Ark*. Encino, CA: Shilysca Press, 2005.

Zeltzer, Paul: *Brain Tumors: Leaving the Garden of Eden*. Encino, CA: Shilysca Press, 2004.

SERIES BOOKS BASED ON THERAPY PROGRAM

Kendall, Philip C.: *Coping Cat Workbook*. Ardmore, PA: Workbook Publishing, 1992.
Based on a program of 16 therapy sessions promoting coping skills for dealing with anxiety. A *Coping Cat Notebook* is also provided with each workbook so that each child can write journal entries for each assignment.

Kendall, Philip C., Muniya Choudhury, Jennifer Hudson, and Alicia Webb: *The C.A.T. Project Workbook for the Cognitive Behavioral Treatment of Anxious Adolescents*. Ardmore, PA: Workbook Publishing, 1992.
Based on a program of 16 sessions for individual cognitive-behavioral therapy (CBT) for anxiety in older adolescents (14 to 17 years of age), using a workbook format.

Kendall, Philip C.: *Stop and Think Workbook*, 2nd ed. Ardmore, PA: Workbook Publishing, 1992.
Based on a program of 20 therapy sessions that provide opportunities to teach children to be less impulsive. Activities in the workbook teach children to recognize and identify their feelings and learn problem-solving in a variety of situations.

Nelson, W. Michael, and A. J. Finch, Jr.: *Keeping Your Cool: The Anger Management Workbook*. Ardmore, PA: Workbook Publishing, 1996.
Workbook for helping adolescents and preadolescents deal with their anger.

Stark, Kevin, and Philip C. Kendall: *Taking Action: A Workbook for Overcoming Depression*. Ardmore, PA: Workbook Publishing, 1996. Based on a program of an 18-session treatment program for use with youth who have depressed mood, dysthymia, or a unipolar depressive disorder. The program can be delivered in either a group or an individual format.

{ APPENDIX D }

Helpful Pain Web Sites

American Academy of Pediatrics: www.aap.org

American Pain Foundation: www.painfoundation.org

American Pain Society: www.ampainsoc.org

Children's Cancer Pain Network: www.childcancerpain.org

Energy healing info: www.reiki.org

General info on medical conditions: www.healingwell.com

General info on pediatric conditions: www.kidshealth.org,
www.keepkidshealthy.com, www.pediatricnetwork.org/
index.htm

General info on pediatric pain: www.pedspain.nursing.uiowa.edu

Iyengar yoga: www.bksiyengar.com

Meditation info: www.innerkidz.org, www.insightla.org, and www.braveheart.org

National Childhood Cancer Foundation: www.nccf.org

National Council for Headache Education: www.achenet.org/kids

Pediatric Pain e-mail list-serve: www.pediatric-pain.ca

Society for Developmental and Behavioral Pediatrics: www.sdbp.org

UCLA Pediatric Pain Program: www.healthcare.ucla.edu/pedspain

{ INDEX }